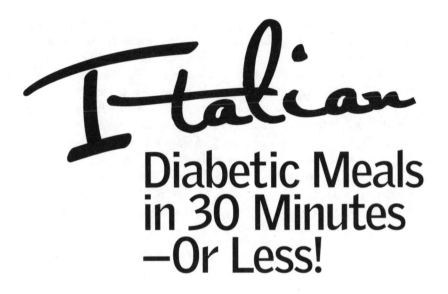

Italian
Diabetic Meals in 30 Minutes —Or Less!

Robyn Webb

American Diabetes Association®

Cure • Care • Commitment®

Director, Book Publishing, John Fedor; *Associate Director, Consumer Books,* Sherrye Landrum; *Editor,* Rebecca Lanning; *Composition,* Circle Graphics, Inc.; *Cover Design,* Koncept, Inc. *Printer,* Port City Press, Inc.

Printed in the United States of America
1 3 5 7 9 10 8 6 4 2

The suggestions and information contained in this publication are generally consistent with the *Clinical Practice Recommendations* and other policies of the American Diabetes Association, but they do not represent the policy or position of the Association or any of its boards or committees. Reasonable steps have been taken to ensure the accuracy of the information presented. However, the American Diabetes Association cannot ensure the safety or efficacy of any product or service described in this publication. Individuals are advised to consult a physician or other appropriate health care professional before undertaking any diet or exercise program or taking any medication referred to in this publication. Professionals must use and apply their own professional judgment, experience, and training and should not rely solely on the information contained in this publication before prescribing any diet, exercise, or medication. The American Diabetes Association—its officers, directors, employees, volunteers, and members—assumes no responsibility or liability for personal or other injury, loss, or damage that may result from the suggestions or information in this publication.

♾ The paper in this publication meets the requirements of the ANSI Standard Z39.48-1992 (permanence of paper).

ADA titles may be purchased for business or promotional use or for special sales. To purchase this book in large quantities, or for custom editions of this book with your logo, contact Lee Romano Sequeira, Special Sales & Promotions, at the address below, or at LRomano@diabetes.org or 703-299-2046.

American Diabetes Association
1701 North Beauregard Street
Alexandria, Virginia 22311

Library of Congress Cataloging-in-Publication Data
Webb, Robyn.
   Italian diabetic meals in 30 minutes—or less! / Robyn Webb.
      p. cm.
   Includes bibliographical references and index.
   ISBN 1-58040-220-8 (alk. paper)
   1. Diabetes—Diet therapy—Recipes. 2. Cookery, Italian. 3. Quick and easy cookery. I. Title.

RC662.W3557 2005
641.5'6314—dc22
                      2004029041

*This book is lovingly dedicated
to all my readers,
who know that 30 minutes in the kitchen
can produce hours of eating pleasure!*

Contents

Acknowledgments

It's always a team effort to produce a book, and this book is no exception. My thanks go out to Sherrye Landrum, who thoroughly believes in the "30 Minutes or Less" concept and saw the need for me to continue that vision. John Fedor has always been a great support, from my very first book, *Diabetic Meals in 30 Minutes—Or Less!*, right up through this one, the seventh that I have written for the American Diabetes Association.

I am grateful to Lyn Wheeler, who is both meticulous and focused as she analyzes recipes for their nutritional content. Her work is more important to me than I think she'll ever know.

I also thank the staff at *Diabetes Forecast* magazine, especially Peter Banks, Andrew Keegan, John Warren, and Marcia Mazur, for their continued support of my work and for sharing my passion for good food.

And, finally, my thanks go out to my friends in Italy, particularly in Tuscany, who inspire me every day. Their deep belief is that the best food is the simplest food, prepared with love and enjoyed with family and friends, and well . . . what can be healthier than that?

Buon Appetito!

Cooking the "30 Minutes or Less" Way

In 1996, when I wrote my first book, *Diabetic Meals in 30 Minutes—Or Less!*, there was a growing need for quick and easy-to-prepare foods. Now that need is insatiable. As I have watched the nine years pass between my first book and this one, I see that people have even less time and the world moves even faster. But my readers still want food that tastes great even with minimal effort. That is what leads me to continue this series, and each year I hope to deliver on the promise that good food can be prepared in minimal time.

The inspiration for this title, *Italian Diabetic Meals in 30 Minutes—Or Less!*, truly does come from the heart. Throughout my travels in Italy, I have found that the Mediterranean life just feels right. Preparation of simple foods enjoyed in the company of one's friends and family is something I strive for right here in my American home. The bold aroma of basil, the juicy ripeness of ruby red tomatoes, the purity of golden olive oil, and the ocean-fresh taste of seafood can be staples in your own home kitchen, and you don't have to spend hours and hours of your precious time to prepare daily meals.

For people with diabetes, the scientific evidence points more and more to the benefits of a Mediterranean-style food program. While more research is underway, the logic makes sense. Olive oil is a good source of monounsaturated fat, and the abundance of fruits and vegetables, lean meats, fresh seafood, and whole grains touted on this kind of plan leads to a healthy heart and a healthy weight.

You will notice that almost all the recipes require only one pan, usually a standard 10- or 12-inch skillet. This significantly reduces the amount of cleanup necessary and should be factored into your overall time. The ingredient lists are relatively short and use common items found in every major market across the country. These factors also figure prominently in the "30 Minutes or Less" concept. In Mediterranean kitchens, most home cooks also use a minimal amount of equipment.

To keep within the time frame, please note that you should read the recipe thoroughly before you start preparing. Make sure all ingredients are out and ready to go. Always begin by preparing everything that needs to be sliced, chopped, or diced, even the garnish. With all your knife work out of the way, cooking is streamlined and simple. And speaking of knives, I highly recommend that you check with a local cookware store about receiving professional lessons in knife skills. My knife skills class is one of my most popular cooking classes and with good reason. The more you know about using your knife efficiently, the faster cooking goes. When cooking doesn't bog you down, you can get to other healthy activities, like exercising!

I hope you enjoy this new collection of recipes, which have been specially designed to help you cook quickly and control your blood sugar, your weight, and other factors important in diabetes management. Indeed, some of my Italian friends control their diabetes solely through diet and exercise. They are truly inspiring to me, and they never sacrifice good flavor to manage their diabetes. In fact, the opposite is true: the good, pure, and true tastes of the food help them stay on the path of healthy living.

Enjoy and mangia!

Ciao,
Robyn Webb

Notes on Ingredients

First and foremost you should relax in the comfort of knowing that you need not run to any specialty stores for any of the ingredients in this book, unless you really want to. You should be able to find everything you need at your local market. Once in a while, however, consider shopping at a farmer's market or even growing a few fresh herbs or perhaps your own tomatoes. Even if you live in a city as I do, you can successfully turn your small outdoor deck or front step into a mini garden redolent with the heady aromas of fresh produce.

Here are some notes on some of the ingredients in this book. Although they are common ingredients, I have provided a few extra details to ensure that you get the maximum flavor in every bite!

Olive Oil

Called "liquid gold" in Italy, olive oil is one of the most misunderstood ingredients in cooking. Extra virgin olive oil comes from the first pressing of the olives and is considered to have the finest taste. Its low acidity and smoothness make it shine when used in salad dressings or for dipping bread. While you can certainly use one type of olive oil for all your needs, you might like to save your dollars and purchase an inexpensive olive oil for cooking and then splurge a bit on a better olive oil when you really can taste it, such as in salads. There are hundreds of olive oils to choose from, and the decision remains a personal one. I have tried many olive oils on the market, and I continue to find new favorites.

How you store your olive oil does make a difference. To make sure your olive oil stays fresh, keep it in a dark or opaque container where the light and air cannot penetrate it deeply. Try to use your olive oil within a year so that it doesn't become rancid. Unlike wine, olive oils do not improve with age.

We know that olive oil is an excellent source of monounsaturated fat, the kind of fat that is good for your heart. Follow the advice of your physician or registered dietitian to incorporate a little of the liquid gold into your food plan.

Herbs and Spices

Throughout this book I have listed fresh and dried herbs and various spices for the recipes. Sometimes the recipe works better with the dried ingredients, but where noted you can easily exchange the two. If you use dried herbs and spices, please make sure that they are as fresh as they can be. The shelf life for best cooking results is one year on dried herbs and spices. After that, the essential oils begin to dissipate and the flavor declines. Store all your dried herbs and spices away from heat and light and check on them often to ensure their freshness.

I am no gardener, and I say that with good reason. But anyone can grow fresh herbs! You don't have to have two green thumbs (last time I checked, my thumbs had no green hue at all!). I highly recommend that you grow herbs even if you have limited outdoor space. All it takes is one plant to get things going, some good soil, sun, water, and a little love. Pick off what you need for a recipe and let the aromas of the herbs scent your outdoor living space. All my friends in Italy grow their own herbs; it's an act of love for them.

Tomatoes

When a recipe calls for fresh tomatoes, use the recipe only when tomatoes are in season, from late spring to late summer. After that, just skip the recipe. In most parts of the U.S., fresh tomatoes are not flavorful all year round. I am very much a seasonal cook, and you will enjoy your food many times over if you stick to seasonal cooking.

When shopping for tomatoes, look for the reddest, firmest tomatoes you can find. If you can locate them, the heirloom tomatoes that make their way to major supermarkets are particularly nice. For the very best results, find a farmer's market and get your tomatoes there. They often have the best selection. Never store you tomatoes anywhere but on the kitchen counter. Never place tomatoes in the refrigerator because the chill dissipates the flavor dramatically.

For canned tomatoes, consider buying them whole and crushing them in your hand, a traditional way I was taught in Italy. In fact, I look forward to digging my hand in the can and crushing the tomatoes between my fingers. Talk about a sensory experience! You should look for canned whole plum tomatoes. Already diced tomatoes are perfectly fine, but just try crushing the whole ones yourself every now and then.

Garlic

There is no substitute for fresh garlic. I will always state that you should use fresh garlic. My friends in Italy would never use anything else. It takes no time to chop up and the results are worth it. I have never quite understood the appeal of already chopped garlic. I know it's quick, but talk about a lack of flavor! So what if your hands smell like garlic! At least you put a little love into the process by getting close to the food. It always strikes me as too "sanitary" to use the premade stuff.

Store your garlic at room temperature and try to use it within at least a week or two. If it shows signs of sprouting, it can taste bitter and you should discard it.

Fresh Meats and Seafood

This book contains mostly main dish ideas. For the freshest meat, plan on buying it and cooking it soon thereafter. There's nothing wrong with freezing meats and seafood for future use, but I prefer to cook as freshly as possible.

Consider buying organic meats and seafood for the taste alone. I have no evidence that you'll live a longer and healthier life because you eat organically, but the taste of organic meats and seafood is outstanding.

Use meats and poultry within 48 hours or a maximum 72 hours after purchase. Use seafood within 24 hours for best results. If you do freeze any meats, poultry, or seafood, make sure you wrap it in heavy-duty butcher or freezer paper and then place it in a Ziploc freezer bag. Freeze meats and poultry no more than 5–6 months and seafood no more than 3 months for best results. Never thaw any animal products at room temperature. Always place them in a refrigerator to thaw.

Cheeses

It wouldn't be Italian cooking if I didn't include some cheese! You will notice, however, that I mostly use highly concentrated cheeses that don't require you to add copious amounts to get flavor. I use some Parmesan, mozzarella, and goat cheeses, but just enough to enhance the taste of the dish and certainly less than what might be served in a restaurant. You might make an exception and shop at a specialty store for the finest cheeses. Remember that you are using them to add a bold dash of flavor, so they have to be good!

Cheese is source of saturated fat, so please check with your physician or dietitian about how to fit it into your food plan.

There you have it—a few words on the ingredients you will need. It is not a long list, but it is an important one. An Italian friend of mine once said that nothing is more important than the quality of your food. Americans, he said, concentrate too much on quantity and miss the point of healthy eating entirely.

I couldn't agree more.

The Main Dishes

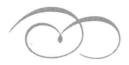

Fish (Pesce)

Baked Cod with Fresh Tomato Topping

4 Servings / Serving Size: 4 oz

1/2 Tbsp olive oil
1 small shallot, minced
1/2 clove garlic, minced
3 medium plum tomatoes, chopped

1 Tbsp minced basil
Salt and pepper to taste
1 lb cod filets
1/2 Tbsp butter
1 Tbsp lemon juice

1 Preheat the oven to 375 degrees.

2 Heat the oil in a small skillet over medium heat and sauté the shallot and garlic until tender, about 1–2 minutes. Add the tomatoes, basil, salt, and pepper and bring to a boil. Simmer, uncovered, for 2 minutes.

3 Meanwhile, arrange the cod filets in 4 individual au gratin dishes. Dot with butter and lemon juice and spread the tomato mixture on top.

4 Bake for 15 minutes or until the fish is opaque.

Exchanges
1 Vegetable
3 Very Lean Meat
1/2 Fat

Calories 143
  Calories from Fat . . . 37
Total Fat . . . . 4 g
  Saturated Fat . . . . . 1.3 g
Cholesterol . . . . 52 mg
Sodium . . . . 88 mg
Total Carbohydrate . . 5 g
  Dietary Fiber . . . . 1 g
  Sugars . . . . 3 g
Protein . . . . 21 g

Broiled Tuna with Cherry Tomato Sauce

4 Servings / Serving Size: 4 oz

3 tsp olive oil
1/2 cup diced onion
3 garlic cloves, minced
3 cups cherry tomatoes, halved
1/2 cup dry red wine
1 Tbsp balsamic vinegar
5 black olives, halved
2 tsp capers
1/4 cup chopped basil leaves
4 4-oz tuna steaks
Salt and pepper

1 Heat 2 tsp of the oil in a large skillet over medium heat. Add the onion and garlic and sauté for 4 minutes. Add the cherry tomatoes and sauté for 2 minutes. Add the wine and balsamic vinegar and bring to a boil. Lower the heat and simmer for 3 minutes. Add the olives, capers, and basil and cook 1 minute.

2 Preheat the oven broiler. Place the tuna on a broiler pan. Brush with the remaining 1 tsp of olive oil, and sprinkle with salt and pepper. Broil the tuna for about 4 minutes per side or until done as desired. Serve the tuna with the cherry tomato sauce.

Exchanges

2 Vegetable
3 Very Lean Meat
2 Fat

Calories 247
  Calories from Fat . . . 88
Total Fat . . . . 10 g
  Saturated Fat . . . . . 1.9 g
Cholesterol . . . . 42 mg
Sodium . . . . 146 mg
Total Carbohydrate . . 9 g
  Dietary Fiber . . . . 2 g
  Sugars . . . . 6 g
Protein . . . . 27 g

Cod with Grilled Tomatoes

4 Servings / Serving Size: 4 oz

2 red tomatoes, cut into 4 slices each
    Salt and fresh ground pepper to taste
1 lb cod filets, about 1 inch thick
2 Tbsp olive oil, divided
2 tsp Dijon mustard
1 Tbsp minced shallots
2 Tbsp lemon juice

1 Preheat the oven broiler. Place the tomato slices on a foil-lined broiler pan. Sprinkle with salt and pepper. Broil 2 inches from the heat source for 2 minutes. Remove from the broiler.

2 Sprinkle the cod filets with additional salt and pepper to taste. Heat 1 Tbsp of the oil in a large skillet over medium-high heat. Add the cod filets and sauté on each side for about 5 minutes. Remove from the pan.

3 Set each cod filet over 2 slices of tomato. Combine the remaining 1 Tbsp of olive oil, mustard, shallots, and lemon juice. Sprinkle over each cod filet.

Exchanges
1 Vegetable
3 Very Lean Meat
1 Fat

Calories	174
Calories from Fat	71
Total Fat	8 g
Saturated Fat	1.1 g
Cholesterol	49 mg
Sodium	137 mg
Total Carbohydrate	5 g
Dietary Fiber	1 g
Sugars	2 g
Protein	21 g

Cod with Oregano and Lemon

4 Servings / Serving Size: 4 oz

4 4-oz cod filets
3/4 tsp dried oregano
1 Tbsp olive oil
3 garlic cloves, finely minced
1 Tbsp lemon juice
Salt and pepper to taste

1 Preheat the oven to 400 degrees. Arrange the cod filets in a baking pan. Rub each filet with oregano. Sprinkle with olive oil, garlic, lemon juice, salt, and pepper.

2 Bake the fish, uncovered, for about 15 minutes, until it is cooked through but tender.

Exchanges
3 Very Lean Meat
1/2 Fat

Calories 127
  Calories from Fat . . . 37
Total Fat . . . . 4 g
  Saturated Fat . . . . . 0.6 g
Cholesterol . . . . 49 mg
Sodium . . . . 70 mg
Total Carbohydrate . . 1 g
  Dietary Fiber . . . . 0 g
  Sugars . . . . 1 g
Protein . . . . 20 g

Flounder with Red Pepper Sauce

4 Servings / Serving Size: 4–5 oz

- **2** cloves garlic, minced
- **2** jarred roasted red peppers,
  coarsely chopped
- **2** Tbsp toasted walnuts
- **1** Tbsp freshly grated
  Parmesan cheese
- **1 1/2** Tbsp olive oil
- **4** 4-5-oz flounder filets
  Salt and pepper to taste

1 In a food processor, combine the garlic, roasted red peppers, walnuts, and cheese. Pulse until combined. Slowly add the olive oil and continue to mix until smooth.

2 Preheat the oven broiler. Place the flounder on a broiler pan lined with foil. Sprinkle with salt and pepper. Broil for 6–7 minutes until cooked through.

3 Warm the sauce in a small saucepan. Serve the sauce with the swordfish.

Exchanges
3 Very Lean Meat
1 1/2 Fat

Calories	184
Calories from Fat	84
Total Fat	9 g
Saturated Fat	1.5 g
Cholesterol	61 mg
Sodium	125 mg
Total Carbohydrate	2 g
Dietary Fiber	0 g
Sugars	1 g
Protein	23 g

Grilled Salmon with Fresh Tomato Sauce

4 Servings / Serving Size: 4 oz

2 tsp olive oil
4 ripe tomatoes, seeded and diced
2 tsp capers
1 tsp fresh chopped oregano
1 tsp fresh chopped thyme
4 4-oz salmon filets

1 Heat the olive oil in a large skillet over medium-high heat. Add the tomatoes to the skillet and sauté for 3 minutes. Add the capers and herbs and continue to cook for 4 minutes. Season with salt and pepper.

2 Meanwhile, preheat the oven broiler and spray a foil-lined broiler pan with cooking spray. Place the salmon on the tray and broil 4–6 inches from the heat source for 8–10 minutes. To serve, spoon some sauce onto each plate. Top with the salmon filet.

Exchanges
1 Vegetable
3 Lean Meat
1 Fat

Calories 241
 Calories from Fat . . 112
Total Fat . . . . 12 g
 Saturated Fat . . . . . 2.0 g
Cholesterol . . . . 77 mg
Sodium . . . . 113 mg
Total Carbohydrate . . 7 g
 Dietary Fiber . . . . 2 g
 Sugars . . . . 4 g
Protein . . . . 25 g

Marjoram-Flavored Sole Filets

4 Servings / Serving Size: 4–5 oz

2 tsp olive oil, divided
1 shallot, minced
1 garlic clove, minced
1 small carrot, diced
3 Tbsp dry white wine

1 Tbsp minced fresh marjoram
(2 tsp dried)
Salt and pepper to taste
4 4–5-oz sole filets
2 Tbsp dry bread crumbs

1 Preheat the oven to 400 degrees.

2 Heat 1 tsp of the olive oil in a skillet over medium-high heat. Add the shallot and garlic and sauté for 2 minutes. Add the carrot and sauté for 4 minutes. Add the wine and sauté for 4 minutes. Add the marjoram, salt, and pepper and sauté for 2 minutes.

3 Place the sole filets in a baking dish. Spread the shallot and carrot mixture over the filets.
Combine the remaining olive oil and the bread crumbs. Sprinkle the bread crumbs over the filets.

4 Bake for 8–10 minutes until the top is lightly browned and the fish is cooked through.

Exchanges
1 Vegetable
3 Very Lean Meat
1/2 Fat

Calories 151
  Calories from Fat . . . 34
Total Fat . . . . 4 g
  Saturated Fat . . . . . 0.3 g
Cholesterol . . . . 60 mg
Sodium . . . . 134 mg
Total Carbohydrate . . 5 g
  Dietary Fiber . . . . 1 g
  Sugars . . . . 1 g
Protein . . . . 22 g

Parsley- and Olive-Topped Cod

4 Servings / Serving Size: 4 oz

1/2 cup minced parsley
1/4 cup finely diced celery
  3 Tbsp minced black olives
  2 garlic cloves, finely minced
  2 Tbsp lemon juice
  2 tsp olive oil
  1 tsp dried oregano
    Salt and pepper to taste
    Nonstick cooking spray
  4 4-oz cod filets

1 In a bowl, combine the parsley, celery, olives, garlic, lemon juice, olive oil, and oregano. Season with salt and pepper.

2 Preheat the oven broiler. Spray a foil-lined broiler pan with the cooking spray. Place the cod filets on the pan and broil 4–6 inches from the heat source for 6–7 minutes until cooked through.

3 Serve the cod with the parsley and olive topping.

Exchanges
3 Very Lean Meat
1/2 Fat

Calories 131
  Calories from Fat . . . 37
Total Fat . . . . 4 g
  Saturated Fat . . . . . 0.6 g
Cholesterol . . . . 49 mg
Sodium . . . . 128 mg
Total Carbohydrate . . 2 g
  Dietary Fiber . . . . 1 g
  Sugars . . . . 1 g
Protein . . . . 21 g

Salmon in White Wine and Leeks

4 Servings / Serving Size: 4 oz

2 tsp olive oil
3 leeks, sliced in half, washed, and sliced thin
1/2 onion, chopped
3 garlic cloves, minced

4 4-oz salmon filets
1/3 cup dry white wine
2 Tbsp lemon juice
Salt and pepper to taste
2 Tbsp minced dill

1 Preheat the oven to 350 degrees. Heat the oil in a skillet over medium-high heat. Add the leeks, onion, and garlic and sauté for 5–7 minutes until soft.

2 Tear off 4 squares of heavy-duty aluminum foil large enough to hold the salmon with enough foil left over to fold. Place a piece of salmon in the center of each square. Drizzle the wine and lemon juice evenly over each packet. Spread the leek mixture over each piece of salmon. Season with salt and pepper. Top with dill.

3 Fold the ends of the foil over the salmon to form a packet. Place the packets on a baking sheet and bake for 10–15 minutes until the salmon is tender. To serve, place the foil packets on a plate and unfold.

Exchanges
3 Vegetable
3 Lean Meat
1/2 Fat

Calories 270
 Calories from Fat. . 110
Total Fat . . . . 12 g
 Saturated Fat . . . . . 2.0 g
Cholesterol . . . . 77 mg
Sodium . . . . 75 mg
Total Carbohydrate . 12 g
 Dietary Fiber . . . . 2 g
 Sugars . . . . 5 g
Protein . . . . 26 g

Salmon with Fresh Tomato and Garlic Sauce

4 Servings / Serving Size: 4 oz

2 tsp olive oil, divided
3 garlic cloves, minced
1 small onion, chopped
1/2 cup low-fat, reduced-sodium chicken broth

1 cup halved cherry tomatoes
2 Tbsp pitted, minced black olives
1 Tbsp minced fresh basil
4 4-oz salmon filets

1 Heat 1 tsp of the olive oil in a skillet over medium-high heat. Add the garlic and onion and sauté for 4 minutes.

2 Add the broth, reduce the heat, cover, and simmer for 3 minutes. Stir in the tomatoes, olives, and basil and cook for 2 more minutes.

3 Meanwhile, preheat the oven broiler. Brush the remaining 1 tsp of olive oil over the salmon filets.
Place the filets on a broiler pan 4 inches from the heat source and broil for 8–10 minutes until the fish is cooked through. Serve the salmon with the tomato sauce.

Exchanges
1 Vegetable
3 Lean Meat
1 Fat

Calories	241
Calories from Fat	115
Total Fat	13 g
Saturated Fat	2.1 g
Cholesterol	77 mg
Sodium	156 mg
Total Carbohydrate	5 g
Dietary Fiber	1 g
Sugars	3 g
Protein	25 g

Salmon with Lemon and Oregano

4 Servings / Serving Size: 4 oz

4 4-oz salmon filets
Salt and pepper to taste
Nonstick cooking spray
1 small shallot, finely minced
2 1/2 Tbsp fresh lemon juice
1 Tbsp dry white wine
2 tsp minced fresh oregano (1 tsp dried)
1 tsp butter

1 Sprinkle the salmon filets with salt and pepper.

2 Spray a large skillet with cooking spray and heat to medium high. When the pan is hot, add the salmon in two batches. Sear the salmon on both sides for a total of 8–10 minutes. Remove the salmon from the skillet.

3 Add the minced shallot to the pan drippings and sauté for 3 minutes. Add the lemon juice, white wine, and oregano. Cook for 1 minute. Swirl in the butter until it melts and pour the sauce over the cooked salmon.

Exchanges
3 Lean Meat
1/2 Fat

Calories	208
Calories from Fat	96
Total Fat	11 g
Saturated Fat	2.3 g
Cholesterol	80 mg
Sodium	68 mg
Total Carbohydrate	2 g
Dietary Fiber	0 g
Sugars	0 g
Protein	24 g

Seared Bass with Basil

4 Servings / Serving Size: 4 oz

1 1/2 Tbsp olive oil
   1 lb sea bass filets or any
     other thick firm
     white fish
     Salt and pepper
   4 garlic cloves, thickly sliced
1/4 tsp red pepper flakes

   1 15-oz can diced tomatoes,
     drained
   8 whole basil leaves
1/4 tsp dried oregano
   2 Tbsp balsamic vinegar
   2 tsp sugar

1 Heat the oil in a large nonstick skillet over medium heat. Sprinkle the fish filets with salt and pepper. Sear the fish for 3 minutes per side. Remove from the skillet.

2 Add the garlic and red pepper flakes to the skillet and sauté 30 seconds. Add the tomatoes, basil, and oregano and bring to a boil. Put the fish back in the pan and cook for 7 minutes until it barely flakes.

3 In a small saucepan, combine the vinegar and sugar and cook for 2 minutes until syrupy. To serve, place the tomato basil sauce on each plate. Top with the fish. Drizzle the vinegar and sugar mixture over each filet.

Exchanges
1 Vegetable
3 Very Lean Meat
1 Fat

Calories 184
  Calories from Fat. . . 66
Total Fat . . . . 7 g
  Saturated Fat . . . . . 0.7 g
Cholesterol . . . . 47 mg
Sodium . . . . 202 mg
Total Carbohydrate . . 7 g
  Dietary Fiber . . . . 1 g
  Sugars . . . . 6 g
Protein . . . . 22 g

Seared Tuna with Roasted Red Pepper and Basil Sauce

4 Servings / Serving Size: 4 oz

4 4-oz tuna steaks
2 Tbsp lemon juice
Salt and pepper to taste
Nonstick cooking spray

SAUCE
1 7-oz jar roasted red peppers, chopped
1/4 cup lemon juice
2 Tbsp minced fresh basil
1 Tbsp minced fresh parsley
1 1/2 Tbsp olive oil
1 tsp balsamic vinegar
Salt and pepper to taste

1 Combine the tuna with the 2 Tbsp lemon juice, salt, and pepper. Marinate for 10 minutes.

2 Meanwhile, puree half the roasted red peppers in a food processor. Add the puree and the remaining chopped pieces of roasted red pepper to a small saucepan. Add the remaining sauce ingredients to the saucepan. Heat on low and simmer for 5–6 minutes.

3 Meanwhile spray a large non-stick skillet with cooking spray. Heat the skillet on high heat. Add the tuna steaks and sear on both sides until done as desired: 4 minutes for rare; 7 minutes for medium; or 10 minutes for well done.

4 Serve the tuna with some of the heated sauce.

Exchanges
1 Vegetable
3 Very Lean Meat
2 Fat

Calories	223
Calories from Fat	95
Total Fat	11 g
Saturated Fat	2.0 g
Cholesterol	42 mg
Sodium	153 mg
Total Carbohydrate	5 g
Dietary Fiber	1 g
Sugars	2 g
Protein	26 g

Swordfish Sicilian Style

4 Servings / Serving Size: 4–5 oz

2 tsp olive oil
4 5-oz swordfish steaks
   (about 1/2 inch thick)
1/2 cup diced onion
2 tsp anchovy paste
2 cups canned crushed
   tomatoes

1 Tbsp tomato paste
2 tsp red wine or balsamic vinegar
1 tsp sugar
1/2 tsp dried rosemary
1 Tbsp capers
1/4 tsp salt
1/4 tsp fresh ground black pepper

1 Heat the oil in a large nonstick skillet over medium-high heat. Add the swordfish steaks and cook on each side for 3–4 minutes. Remove the fish from the skillet.

2 Add the onion and sauté for 3 minutes. Add the anchovy paste and cook for 1 minute. Add the crushed tomatoes, tomato paste, vinegar, sugar, and rosemary and bring to a boil. Lower the heat and simmer for 5–6 minutes. Add the capers, salt, and pepper.

3 Put the fish back in the skillet and simmer for 3–4 minutes. Serve the fish with the sauce.

Exchanges
3 Vegetable
3 Lean Meat
1/2 Fat

Calories 264
  Calories from Fat . . . 77
Total Fat . . . . 9 g
  Saturated Fat . . . . . 2.0 g
Cholesterol . . . . 58 mg
Sodium . . . . 807 mg
Total Carbohydrate . 14 g
  Dietary Fiber . . . . 4 g
  Sugars . . . . 8 g
Protein . . . . 31 g

Swordfish with Garlic and Parsley

4 Servings / Serving Size: 4 oz

4 4-oz swordfish steaks
3 garlic cloves, minced
Juice of 2 lemons
1 1/2 Tbsp olive oil
2 Tbsp minced parsley
Salt and pepper to taste

1 Combine all ingredients and marinate the swordfish for 10 minutes.

2 Preheat the oven broiler. Place the swordfish on a broiler tray lined with foil. Broil the swordfish 6 inches from the heat source for 10 minutes per inch of thickness.

Exchanges
3 Lean Meat

Calories 163
Calories from Fat. . . 63
Total Fat . . . . 7 g
Saturated Fat . . . . . 1.6 g
Cholesterol . . . . 44 mg
Sodium . . . . 104 mg
Total Carbohydrate . . 1 g
Dietary Fiber . . . . 0 g
Sugars . . . . 1 g
Protein . . . . 22 g

Tilapia in Zesty Tomato Sauce

4 Servings / Serving Size: 4 oz

2 tsp olive oil
1 small onion, minced
2 garlic cloves, minced
1 14-oz can diced tomatoes
1 Tbsp minced parsley
1/8–1/4 tsp red pepper flakes
4 4-oz tilapia filets (or red snapper)

1 Heat the oil in a skillet over medium-high heat. Add the onion and garlic and sauté for 3 minutes. Add the tomatoes, parsley, and red pepper flakes. Bring to a boil, lower the heat, and simmer for 5–6 minutes.

2 Meanwhile, preheat the oven broiler. Place the fish filets on a broiler pan and broil 4 inches from the heat source for 7–8 minutes until the fish is cooked through.

3 Serve the fish with the tomato sauce.

Exchanges
1 Vegetable
3 Very Lean Meat
1/2 Fat

Calories 162
 Calories from Fat . . . 45
Total Fat . . . . 5 g
 Saturated Fat . . . . . 1.3 g
Cholesterol . . . . 76 mg
Sodium . . . . 229 mg
Total Carbohydrate . . 7 g
 Dietary Fiber . . . . 2 g
 Sugars . . . . 5 g
Protein . . . . 24 g

Trout with Oven-Broiled Peppers

4 Servings / Serving Size: about 5 oz

4 5-oz trout filets
2 tsp finely chopped rosemary leaves
2 tsp finely minced oregano
1 tsp finely minced thyme
4 tsp lemon juice
2 tsp olive oil
1 red pepper, seeded and sliced into 1-inch strips
1 green pepper, seeded and sliced into 1-inch strips

1 Preheat the oven broiler. Place the trout on a lined baking sheet or broiler pan. Combine the rosemary leaves, oregano, and thyme. Sprinkle the herb mixture over each piece of fish. Sprinkle the trout with lemon juice and oil.

2 Surround the fish with the pepper strips. Broil the fish and peppers together about 5 inches from the heat source for 5–8 minutes until the trout is tender and the peppers are slightly charred.

Exchanges
1 Vegetable
4 Lean Meat

Calories 251
  Calories from Fat . . 107
Total Fat . . . . 12 g
  Saturated Fat . . . . . 2.0 g
Cholesterol . . . . 82 mg
Sodium . . . . 78 mg
Total Carbohydrate . . 5 g
  Dietary Fiber . . . . 2 g
  Sugars . . . . 3 g
Protein . . . . 30 g

Tuna on a Bed of Arugula

4 Servings / Serving Size: 4 oz

Nonstick cooking spray
2 Tbsp olive oil, divided
1 lb tuna, cut into 4 pieces
Salt and pepper to taste
1 lb fresh arugula or spinach, stemmed, washed, and patted dry
1 Tbsp balsamic vinegar

1 Spray a large skillet with cooking spray. Add 1 Tbsp of oil to the pan and heat until sizzling over medium-high heat.

2 Sprinkle the tuna with salt and pepper. Add the tuna and cook for 3–4 minutes per side or until done as desired. Remove the tuna from the skillet and keep warm.

3 Add the remaining oil to the pan. Add the arugula or spinach and sauté for 2–3 minutes until wilted. Add the balsamic vinegar.

4 To serve, place a mound of the arugula on each plate. Top with the tuna.

Exchanges
1 Vegetable
4 Very Lean Meat
2 Fat

Calories	245
Calories from Fat	115
Total Fat	13 g
Saturated Fat	2.4 g
Cholesterol	42 mg
Sodium	71 mg
Total Carbohydrate	5 g
Dietary Fiber	2 g
Sugars	3 g
Protein	28 g

Tuna Puttanesca

4 Servings / Serving Size: 4–5 oz

Nonstick cooking spray
2 tsp olive oil, divided
4 5-oz tuna steaks
Salt and pepper to taste
1/2 large onion, chopped
3 garlic cloves
1 15-oz can diced tomatoes, undrained
1 tsp anchovy paste
2 tsp capers
2 Tbsp pitted, chopped olives
2 Tbsp dry white wine

1 Spray a large skillet with cooking spray. Add 1 tsp of the olive oil to the pan and heat to medium high.

2 Sprinkle the tuna with salt and pepper. Add the tuna to the pan and sauté for 3–4 minutes per side for medium rare (longer for more well done). Remove the tuna from the pan.

3 Add remaining oil. Add the onion and garlic and sauté for 4 minutes. Add the tomatoes and anchovy paste and bring to a boil. Lower the heat and add the remaining ingredients. Simmer for 5 minutes. Put the tuna back in the sauce, turning once so that the tuna absorbs some of the sauce.

Exchanges
2 Vegetable
4 Very Lean Meat
1 1/2 Fat

Calories 266
 Calories from Fat . . . 90
Total Fat . . . . 10 g
 Saturated Fat . . . . . 2.1 g
Cholesterol . . . . 54 mg
Sodium . . . . 402 mg
Total Carbohydrate . . 9 g
 Dietary Fiber . . . . 2 g
 Sugars . . . . 6 g
Protein . . . . 34 g

Tuna with Currants and Pine Nuts

4 Servings / Serving Size: 4 oz

2 Tbsp currants or raisins
1/2 cup boiling water
2 tsp olive oil
1/2 medium red onion, diced
1 stalk celery, diced
2 garlic cloves, diced

3 Tbsp pine nuts
2 Tbsp minced fresh parsley
Nonstick cooking spray
Salt and pepper to taste
4 4-oz tuna steaks

1 Add the currants or raisins to a bowl. Pour the boiling water over the currants and set aside.

2 Meanwhile, heat the oil in a skillet over medium-high heat. Add the red onion and celery and sauté for 4 minutes. Add the garlic and sauté for 2 minutes. Add the pine nuts and sauté for 2 minutes until they begin to brown. Add the parsley. Drain the currants or raisins and add to the skillet. Cook 1 minute.

3 Preheat the oven broiler. Spray a foil-lined broiler pan with cooking spray. Place the tuna steaks in the pan, sprinkle with salt and pepper, and broil 4–6 inches from the heat source for 6–7 minutes, longer for more well done.

4 Serve the tuna with the currant and pine nut mixture spooned on top of each piece.

Exchanges
1/2 Carbohydrate
4 Very Lean Meat
1 1/2 Fat

Calories 242
  Calories from Fat . . 103
Total Fat . . . . 11 g
  Saturated Fat . . . . . 2.4 g
Cholesterol . . . . 42 mg
Sodium . . . . 55 mg
Total Carbohydrate . . 7 g
  Dietary Fiber . . . . 1 g
  Sugars . . . . 5 g
Protein . . . . 28 g

Tuna with Garlic and Basil

4 Servings / Serving Size: 4 oz

4 4-oz tuna steaks
Salt and pepper to taste
Nonstick cooking spray
2 Tbsp olive oil, divided
3 garlic cloves, minced

2 Tbsp low-fat, reduced-sodium
chicken broth
1 Tbsp balsamic vinegar
1 Tbsp minced fresh basil

1 Sprinkle the tuna with salt and pepper.

2 Spray a large skillet with cooking spray. Heat half of the oil in the skillet over high heat. Add the tuna and sear for 4 minutes per side or until done as desired. Set aside and keep warm.

3 Add the remaining oil and the garlic to the pan and sauté for 30 seconds. Add the broth and vinegar and cook 1 minute. Add the basil.

4 Drizzle the garlic and basil sauce over the cooked tuna.

Exchanges
4 Very Lean Meat
2 Fat

Calories 223
  Calories from Fat . . 109
Total Fat . . . . 12 g
  Saturated Fat . . . . . 2.3 g
Cholesterol . . . . 42 mg
Sodium . . . . 59 mg
Total Carbohydrate . . 2 g
  Dietary Fiber . . . . 0 g
  Sugars . . . . 1 g
Protein . . . . 26 g

Tuna with Pepper Ragu

4 Servings / Serving Size: 4 oz

2 tsp olive oil, divided
2 garlic cloves, minced
1 small onion, diced
1 small red pepper, seeded, cored, and sliced into strips
1 small green pepper, seeded, cored, and sliced into strips

1 15-oz can crushed plum tomatoes
1 Tbsp minced fresh basil
2 tsp dried oregano
Salt and pepper to taste
4 4-oz tuna steaks

1 Heat 1 tsp of the oil in a large skillet over medium-high heat. Add the garlic and onion and sauté for 4 minutes. Add the peppers and sauté for 4 minutes. Add the tomatoes and bring to a boil. Lower the heat and simmer for 5 minutes.

2 Add the basil and oregano and simmer for 5 minutes. Season with salt and pepper.

3 Meanwhile, heat the remaining olive oil on medium-high heat in another nonstick skillet. Sear the tuna on both sides for 6–8 minutes, or longer for well-done tuna.

4 Serve the sauce with the tuna.

Exchanges
3 Vegetable
3 Very Lean Meat
1 1/2 Fat

Calories 244
  Calories from Fat . . . 72
Total Fat . . . . 8 g
  Saturated Fat . . . . . 1.7 g
Cholesterol . . . . 42 mg
Sodium . . . . 339 mg
Total Carbohydrate . 14 g
  Dietary Fiber . . . . 4 g
  Sugars . . . . 9 g
Protein . . . . 28 g

Turbot with Tomatoes and Olives

4 Servings / Serving Size: 4 oz

1 Tbsp olive oil, divided	1/3 cup low-fat, reduced-sodium chicken broth
1/2 cup chopped onion	
2 tsp bottled minced garlic	1/4 cup black olives, pitted
4 4-oz turbot filets	1 cup diced canned tomatoes, drained
1/2 tsp salt	
1/4 tsp black pepper	1 Tbsp chopped fresh basil
1 cup dry white wine	

1 Heat half the olive oil in a nonstick skillet over medium-high heat. Add the onion and garlic and sauté for 3 minutes. Remove from the skillet.

2 Season the turbot filets with salt and pepper. Add the remaining oil to the skillet. Add the turbot filets and cook on each side for 4–5 minutes.

3 Add back the sautéed onion and garlic and then add the wine and broth, cover the pan, and cook for 3 minutes. Add the olives, tomatoes, and basil and cook, covered, for 2 minutes. Serve the fish with the sauce.

Exchanges
1 Vegetable
3 Lean Meat

Calories 199
  Calories from Fat . . . 70
Total Fat . . . . 8 g
  Saturated Fat . . . . . 1.2 g
Cholesterol . . . . 55 mg
Sodium . . . . 711 mg
Total Carbohydrate . . 6 g
  Dietary Fiber . . . . . . 1 g
  Sugars . . . . 4 g
Protein . . . . 19 g

Tuscan Tuna Salad

4 Servings / Serving Size: 3–4 oz

1 small red onion, chopped
1/4 cup minced fresh basil
1/4 cup minced jarred roasted red peppers
1 Tbsp capers
2 Tbsp olive oil
2 Tbsp fresh lemon juice
2 7-oz cans water-packed tuna, drained

Combine all ingredients. Refrigerate for a half hour before serving.

Exchanges
3 Very Lean Meat
1 1/2 Fat

Calories 174
Calories from Fat . . . 68
Total Fat . . . . 8 g
Saturated Fat . . . . . 1.1 g
Cholesterol . . . . 26 mg
Sodium . . . . 381 mg
Total Carbohydrate . . 3 g
Dietary Fiber . . . . 1 g
Sugars . . . . 1 g
Protein . . . . 23 g

Shellfish (Frutti di Mare)

Garlic Shrimp

4 Servings / Serving Size: 4 oz

1 Tbsp olive oil
5 garlic cloves, finely minced
1 lb peeled and deveined large shrimp
(order ahead and have it deveined for you)
3 Tbsp dry white wine
1/2 tsp dried basil
1/4 tsp dried oregano
1 tsp butter, cut into bits

Heat the oil in a large skillet over medium-high heat. Add the garlic and
sauté for 20 seconds. Add the shrimp and cook for 2–3 minutes until they
turn pink. Add the wine, basil, and oregano and cook for 1 minute. Add
the butter and swirl into the sauce until melted.

Exchanges
3 Very Lean Meat
1 Fat

Calories 137
 Calories from Fat . . . 48
Total Fat . . . . 5 g
 Saturated Fat . . . . . 1.3 g
Cholesterol . . . . 177 mg
Sodium . . . . 209 mg
Total Carbohydrate . . 1 g
 Dietary Fiber . . . . 0 g
 Sugars . . . . 1 g
Protein . . . . 19 g

Garlicky Shrimp and Broccoli

4 Servings / Serving Size: 4 oz

2 tsp olive oil
4 garlic cloves, thinly sliced
1/2 small onion, minced
1 lb peeled and deveined large shrimp
    (order ahead and have it deveined for you)
1/2 tsp dried basil
1/2 tsp dried oregano
2 cups broccoli florets
1/3 cup low-fat, reduced-sodium chicken broth
    Salt and pepper to taste
2 Tbsp freshly grated Parmesan cheese

1 Heat the oil in a large skillet over medium-high heat. Add the garlic and onion and sauté for 1 minute.

2 Add the shrimp and sauté for 2 minutes. Add the basil, oregano, and broccoli. Stir to mix. Add the broth, cover, and cook for 2–3 minutes until the broccoli is bright green but tender.

3 Season with salt and pepper. Sprinkle Parmesan cheese over each serving.

Exchanges
1 Vegetable
3 Very Lean Meat
1/2 Fat

Calories	135
Calories from Fat	38
Total Fat	4 g
Saturated Fat	1.0 g
Cholesterol	164 mg
Sodium	260 mg
Total Carbohydrate	4 g
Dietary Fiber	1 g
Sugars	3 g
Protein	20 g

Grilled Parmigiana Shrimp over Sautéed Spinach

4 Servings / Serving Size: 4 oz

2 tsp olive oil, divided
4 garlic cloves, minced
1 lb peeled and deveined large shrimp (order ahead and have it deveined for you)
1/4 cup dry white wine

5 cups spinach leaves, washed and stemmed
Salt and pepper to taste
2 Tbsp freshly grated Parmesan cheese

1 Heat 1 tsp of the olive oil in a large skillet. Add the garlic and shrimp and sauté for 2–3 minutes. Add the wine and sauté for 1 minute until the wine is evaporated.

2 Remove the shrimp from the skillet. Add the remaining 1 tsp of oil. Add the spinach and sauté for 2–3 minutes until it is wilted but before it begins to release its own juices. Season the spinach with salt and pepper and remove it from the skillet.

3 Preheat the oven broiler. Place the shrimp on a broiler pan and sprinkle with Parmesan cheese. Broil in the oven for 1 minute. To serve, place the spinach on a plate and top with the shrimp.

Exchanges
2 Very Lean Meat
1 Fat

Calories	117
Calories from Fat	36
Total Fat	4 g
Saturated Fat	1.0 g
Cholesterol	133 mg
Sodium	204 mg
Total Carbohydrate	2 g
Dietary Fiber	1 g
Sugars	1 g
Protein	16 g

Herbed Scallops

4 Servings / Serving Size: 4 oz

1 lb sea scallops
   Salt and pepper to taste
2 tsp olive oil
3 Tbsp dry white wine or low-fat, reduced-sodium chicken broth
1/2 cup diced canned tomatoes, drained
1 Tbsp minced parsley
1 Tbsp minced basil

1 Sprinkle the scallops with salt and pepper. Heat the olive oil in a nonstick pan over medium-high heat. When hot, add the scallops, in batches if necessary, and sauté on both sides for a total of 4 minutes. Remove the scallops from the pan.

2 Add the wine to the pan and scrape up any browned bits. Add the tomatoes, parsley, and basil and lower the heat, simmering for 5 minutes. Add the scallops back to the sauce and heat for 1 minute.

Exchanges
2 Very Lean Meat
1 Fat

Calories	120
Calories from Fat	45
Total Fat	5 g
Saturated Fat	0.8 g
Cholesterol	27 mg
Sodium	195 mg
Total Carbohydrate	3 g
Dietary Fiber	0 g
Sugars	1 g
Protein	14 g

Herbed Spicy Shrimp

4 Servings / Serving Size: 4 oz

1 Tbsp olive oil
1 onion, diced
2 garlic cloves, minced
1 15-oz can diced tomatoes, drained
2 tsp dried oregano
1 tsp dried basil

1/2 tsp dried thyme
1/4 tsp crushed red pepper flakes
    Salt and pepper to taste
1 lb peeled and deveined large shrimp (order ahead and have it deveined for you)
1 Tbsp minced parsley

1 Heat the olive oil in a large skillet over medium-high heat. Add the onion and garlic and sauté for 4 minutes. Add the tomatoes, oregano, basil, thyme, crushed red pepper flakes, salt, and pepper and bring to a boil. Lower the heat and simmer for 5 minutes.

2 Add the shrimp, cover, and cook over medium heat for 2–3 minutes until the shrimp is cooked through. Top with minced parsley.

Exchanges
1 Vegetable
2 Very Lean Meat
1 Fat

Calories 143
  Calories from Fat. . . 41
Total Fat . . . . 5 g
  Saturated Fat . . . . . 0.7 g
Cholesterol . . . . 161 mg
Sodium . . . . 310 mg
Total Carbohydrate . . 7 g
  Dietary Fiber . . . . 2 g
  Sugars . . . . 5 g
Protein . . . . 19 g

Lemon Scallops with Shallot Sauce

4 Servings / Serving Size: 4 oz

1 lb sea scallops
(halve if very large)
1 Tbsp all-purpose flour
Salt and pepper to taste
1 Tbsp olive oil
1 tsp butter

1/4 cup dry white wine
2 small shallots, minced
1 garlic clove, minced
1 Tbsp lemon juice
1/4 cup minced parsley

1 In a zippered bag, combine the scallops with the flour, salt, and pepper. Shake off excess flour.

2 Heat the oil in a large nonstick skillet over medium-high heat. Add the scallops and sauté for 2–3 minutes per side. Remove the scallops from the skillet.

3 Add the butter, wine, shallots, and garlic to the skillet and sauté for about 2 minutes. Add the lemon juice and cook for 1 minute. Put the scallops back in the skillet and sprinkle with parsley. Serve over rice or noodles.

Exchanges
1/2 Carbohydrate
2 Very Lean Meat
1 Fat

Calories	154
Calories from Fat	64
Total Fat	7 g
Saturated Fat	1.5 g
Cholesterol	30 mg
Sodium	169 mg
Total Carbohydrate	6 g
Dietary Fiber	1 g
Sugars	1 g
Protein	15 g

Scallops Florentine

4 Servings / Serving Size: 4 oz

1 10-oz package frozen spinach, thawed and drained well
4 oz fat-free cream cheese
1/4 tsp nutmeg
    Salt and pepper to taste
1 lb bay scallops, rinsed and patted dry
2 Tbsp fresh lemon juice
1/2 Tbsp butter

1 Preheat the oven to 425 degrees. Combine the spinach, cream cheese, nutmeg, salt, and pepper. Beat well.

2 Place the spinach mixture in the bottom of four individual au gratin dishes. Top with scallops.

3 Sprinkle with lemon juice and dot with butter. Cover with foil and bake for 10 minutes.

Exchanges
1/2 Carbohydrate
3 Very Lean Meat
1/2 Fat

Calories 145
  Calories from Fat . . . 38
Total Fat . . . . 4 g
  Saturated Fat . . . . . 1.4 g
Cholesterol . . . . 34 mg
Sodium . . . . 365 mg
Total Carbohydrate . . 7 g
  Dietary Fiber . . . . 2 g
  Sugars . . . . 1 g
Protein . . . . 20 g

Seafood Mélange

4 Servings / Serving Size: 4 oz

2 tsp olive oil
1 medium onion, chopped
1 slice pancetta, diced
3 garlic cloves, minced
1 15-oz can diced tomatoes, drained

2 tsp tomato paste
2 tsp balsamic vinegar
2 Tbsp minced parsley
1/2 lb peeled and deveined shrimp
1/2 lb sea scallops

1 Heat the olive oil in a large saucepan over medium-high heat. Add the onion and pancetta and sauté for 5 minutes. Add the garlic and sauté for 2 minutes. Add the tomatoes, tomato paste, and balsamic vinegar.

2 Simmer the sauce for 3 minutes. Add the parsley, shrimp, and scallops. Cover the skillet and steam for 3 minutes until the shrimp turns pink and the scallops are cooked through.

Exchanges
2 Vegetable
2 Very Lean Meat
1 Fat

Calories 157
  Calories from Fat . . . 52
Total Fat . . . . 6 g
  Saturated Fat . . . . . 1.2 g
Cholesterol . . . . 98 mg
Sodium . . . . 387 mg
Total Carbohydrate . . 9 g
  Dietary Fiber . . . . 2 g
  Sugars . . . . 5 g
Protein . . . . 18 g

Shrimp and Basil Salad

4 Servings / Serving Size: 4 oz

1 lb cooked, peeled, and deveined large shrimp
2 small zucchini, julienned
1 carrot, julienned
1/2 cup coarsely chopped fresh basil
1 cup halved cherry tomatoes

DRESSING
Juice of 2 limes
1 1/2 Tbsp olive oil
1/2 tsp Dijon mustard
Salt and pepper

1 In a salad bowl, combine the shrimp, zucchini, carrot, basil, and cherry tomatoes.

2 Combine the dressing ingredients. Add the dressing to the shrimp salad and toss. Cover and refrigerate for a half hour before serving.

Exchanges
1 Vegetable
2 Very Lean Meat
1 Fat

Calories 155
  Calories from Fat . . . 56
Total Fat . . . . 6 g
  Saturated Fat . . . . . 0.9 g
Cholesterol . . . . 161 mg
Sodium . . . . 221 mg
Total Carbohydrate . . 6 g
  Dietary Fiber . . . . 2 g
  Sugars . . . . 3 g
Protein . . . . 19 g

Shrimp and Calamari Salad

4 Servings / Serving Size: 4 oz

1/2 lb frozen cooked calamari, thawed and thinly sliced
1/2 lb frozen cooked, peeled, and deveined large shrimp, thawed
2 celery stalks, sliced
2 carrots, thinly sliced
1 small red onion, very thinly sliced
2 Tbsp minced fresh parsley
2 1/2 Tbsp olive oil
2 Tbsp fresh lemon juice
Salt and black pepper to taste

1 Combine the calamari and shrimp in a large bowl. Add the celery, carrots, red onion, and parsley.

2 Whisk together the olive oil and lemon juice. Season with salt and pepper. Add to the seafood and toss well. Serve.

Exchanges
1/2 Carbohydrate
3 Very Lean Meat
2 Fat

Calories 238
  Calories from Fat . . 106
Total Fat . . . . 12 g
  Saturated Fat . . . . . 1.9 g
Cholesterol . . . . 270 mg
Sodium . . . . 394 mg
Total Carbohydrate . . 9 g
  Dietary Fiber . . . . 2 g
  Sugars . . . . 3 g
Protein . . . . 23 g

Chicken (Pollo)

Balsamic Chicken and Tomato

4 Servings / Serving Size: 4 oz

2 tsp olive oil
1 lb boneless, skinless chicken breasts
Salt and pepper to taste
3 scallions, minced
1 cup seeded, chopped plum tomatoes
1/2 cup low-fat, reduced-sodium chicken broth
2 Tbsp balsamic vinegar
Pinch crushed red pepper flakes

1 Heat the olive oil in a nonstick skillet over medium-high heat. Sprinkle the chicken with salt and pepper. Sauté the chicken breasts on both sides for a total of 7–8 minutes. Remove the chicken from the skillet.

2 Add the scallions and sauté for 1 minute. Add the tomatoes and sauté for 2 minutes. Add the broth and bring to a boil. Lower the heat and simmer for 3 minutes. Drizzle in the balsamic vinegar and cook for 2 minutes. Put the chicken back in the skillet and cook for 2 minutes.

Exchanges
1 Vegetable
3 Very Lean Meat
1 Fat

Calories 173
  Calories from Fat . . . 48
Total Fat . . . . 5 g
  Saturated Fat . . . . . 1.1 g
Cholesterol . . . . 69 mg
Sodium . . . . 128 mg
Total Carbohydrate . . 5 g
  Dietary Fiber . . . . 1 g
  Sugars . . . . 3 g
Protein . . . . 26 g

Balsamic Glazed Chicken

4 Servings / Serving Size: 4 oz

4 4-oz boneless, skinless chicken breasts
Salt and pepper to taste
2 tsp dried thyme leaves
1 Tbsp olive oil, divided
2 small shallots, minced
3 Tbsp balsamic vinegar
1/2 cup no-sugar-added raspberry jam

1 Sprinkle the chicken with salt, pepper, and thyme leaves. Heat half the oil in a large nonstick skillet over medium-high heat. Add the chicken and sauté on each side for 4–6 minutes. Remove the chicken from the skillet.

2 Add the remaining oil and the shallots and sauté for 1 minute. Combine the vinegar and jam, add to the skillet, and bring to a boil. Lower the heat and simmer for 2 minutes. Put the chicken and any accumulated juices back in the skillet and simmer for 2 minutes.

Exchanges
1/2 Fruit
4 Very Lean Meat
1 Fat

Calories 199
 Calories from Fat . . . 57
Total Fat . . . . 6 g
 Saturated Fat . . . . . 1.3 g
Cholesterol . . . . 69 mg
Sodium . . . . 61 mg
Total Carbohydrate . . 9 g
 Dietary Fiber . . . . 0 g
 Sugars . . . . 2 g
Protein . . . . 25 g

Broiled Chicken Thighs with Basil and Pepper Sauce

4 Servings / Serving Size: 4 oz

2 tsp olive oil
1 large onion, chopped
1 garlic clove, minced
1 red pepper, cored and diced
1/2 cup torn basil leaves
Salt and pepper to taste
1/4 tsp crushed red pepper
1 lb boneless, skinless chicken thighs
1 Tbsp Parmesan cheese

1 Heat the olive oil in a large skillet over medium heat. Add the onion and sauté for 5 minutes. Add the garlic and the red pepper and sauté for 5 minutes. Add the basil leaves and sauté for 1 minute.

2 Transfer the pepper mixture to a food processor and blend until smooth but somewhat thick. Season with salt, pepper, and crushed red pepper.

3 Preheat the oven broiler. Place the chicken thighs on a broiler pan and broil 6 inches from the heat source, turning once, for a total of 10–12 minutes. Serve the chicken with the sauce and sprinkle with Parmesan cheese.

Exchanges
2 Vegetable
2 Lean Meat
1/2 Fat

Calories	195
Calories from Fat	87
Total Fat	10 g
Saturated Fat	2.4 g
Cholesterol	63 mg
Sodium	65 mg
Total Carbohydrate	8 g
Dietary Fiber	2 g
Sugars	5 g
Protein	19 g

Chicken Cacciatore I

4 Servings / Serving Size: 4 oz

- **2** Tbsp flour
  Salt and pepper to taste
- **1** lb boneless, skinless chicken thighs
- **2** tsp olive oil
- **1** 10-oz package frozen pepper stir fry
- **1** onion, chopped
- **1/3** cup dry red wine
- **2** 15-oz cans diced tomatoes

1 Combine the flour, salt, and pepper. Dredge the chicken in the flour mixture. Heat the oil in a large skillet over medium-high heat. Add the chicken and sauté on both sides for a total of 8–10 minutes. Remove the chicken from the skillet.

2 Add the pepper stir fry and onion and sauté for 4–5 minutes. Add the red wine and tomatoes and bring to a boil. Boil for 3 minutes. Return the chicken to the skillet, lower the heat, and simmer for 3 minutes.

Exchanges
4 Vegetable
3 Lean Meat
1/2 Fat

Calories 293
  Calories from Fat. . 108
Total Fat . . . . 12 g
  Saturated Fat . . . . . 2.9 g
Cholesterol . . . . 81 mg
Sodium . . . . 506 mg
Total Carbohydrate . 19 g
  Dietary Fiber . . . . 5 g
  Sugars . . . . 10 g
Protein . . . . 26 g

Chicken Cacciatore II

4 Servings / Serving Size: 4 oz

4 4-oz boneless, skinless chicken breasts
Salt and pepper to taste
1 1/2 Tbsp olive oil
1 medium onion, chopped
2 garlic cloves, minced
1 tsp chopped fresh rosemary
1 tsp chopped fresh sage
1/2 cup dry white wine
1 28-oz can crushed tomatoes
1/4 cup black olives, pitted

1 Sprinkle the chicken with salt and pepper. Heat the olive oil in a skillet over medium-high heat. Add the chicken breasts, in batches if necessary, to the pan and sauté for 5 minutes per side. Remove the chicken from the skillet.

2 Add the onion and garlic to the skillet and sauté for 3 minutes. Add the herbs and sauté 30 seconds. Add the wine and cook for 2 minutes. Add the tomatoes and bring to a boil. Lower the heat and cook for 8 minutes. Put the chicken breasts back in the skillet and cook for 2 minutes. Add the olives.

Exchanges
4 Vegetable
3 Very Lean Meat
2 Fat

Calories 297
Calories from Fat . . . 87
Total Fat . . . . 10 g
Saturated Fat . . . . . 1.7 g
Cholesterol . . . . 69 mg
Sodium . . . . 675 mg
Total Carbohydrate . 21 g
Dietary Fiber . . . . . . 6 g
Sugars . . . . 13 g
Protein . . . . 29 g

Chicken Cutlets with Garlic Plum Tomato Relish

4 Servings / Serving Size: 4 oz

2 Tbsp flour
Salt and pepper to taste
1 tsp dried rosemary
1 lb boneless, skinless chicken
cutlets
2 tsp olive oil
1/2 cup diced onion

3 garlic cloves, minced
1/3 cup low-fat, reduced-sodium
chicken broth
2 tsp balsamic vinegar
3 plum tomatoes, seeded and
coarsely chopped
1 Tbsp minced parsley

1 Mix together the flour, salt, pepper, and rosemary. Coat the chicken with the flour mixture and shake off the excess. Heat the oil in a large nonstick skillet over medium-high heat. Sauté the chicken for 4 minutes per side and remove it from the skillet.

2 Add the onion and garlic and sauté for 3 minutes. Add the broth and bring to a boil. Reduce the liquid by half. Add the balsamic vinegar and tomatoes and cook for 3 minutes. Add the parsley.

3 Serve the chicken with the relish.

Exchanges
1 Vegetable
4 Very Lean Meat
1/2 Fat

Calories 192
Calories from Fat . . . 49
Total Fat . . . . 5 g
Saturated Fat . . . . . 1.1 g
Cholesterol . . . . 69 mg
Sodium . . . . 107 mg
Total Carbohydrate . . 9 g
Dietary Fiber . . . . 1 g
Sugars . . . . 4 g
Protein . . . . 26 g

Chicken Cutlets with Sun-Dried Tomato Sauce

4 Servings / Serving Size: 4 oz

10 jarred sun-dried tomatoes, plus 2 tsp oil from the jar
4 4-oz boneless, skinless chicken cutlets
1/2 tsp salt
1/4 tsp fresh ground black pepper

2 small shallots, minced
1 cup presliced mushrooms
1/4 cup low-fat, reduced-sodium chicken broth
2 Tbsp dry white wine
1 Tbsp minced parsley

1 Mince the sun-dried tomatoes, reserving 2 tsp of the oil from the jar. Set the tomatoes aside.

2 Sprinkle the chicken with salt and pepper. Heat the reserved oil in a large nonstick skillet over medium-high heat. Add the chicken and cook for 4 minutes per side. Remove the chicken from the pan.

3 Reduce the heat to medium. Add the shallots and sauté for 2 minutes. Add the mushrooms and sauté for 2 minutes. Add the tomatoes, broth, and wine. Boil for 1 minute. Pour the sauce over the chicken and sprinkle with parsley.

Exchanges
1 Vegetable
3 Very Lean Meat
1 Fat

Calories	193
Calories from Fat	60
Total Fat	7 g
Saturated Fat	1.2 g
Cholesterol	69 mg
Sodium	411 mg
Total Carbohydrate	5 g
Dietary Fiber	1 g
Sugars	1 g
Protein	26 g

Chicken in Balsamic Vinegar and Mustard

4 Servings / Serving Size: 4 oz

> **2** tsp olive oil
> **4** 4-oz boneless, skinless chicken breasts
>   Salt and pepper to taste
> **1/2** cup balsamic vinegar
> **1 1/2** Tbsp Dijon mustard
> **1/2** tsp dried thyme
> **1/4** cup toasted pine nuts

1 Heat the olive oil in a large nonstick pan over medium-high heat. Sprinkle the chicken with salt and pepper and sauté the chicken breasts on both sides, for a total of 10 minutes. Remove the chicken from the skillet.

2 Combine the vinegar and mustard and add them to the skillet, scraping up any browned bits. Boil and reduce by a third.

3 Pour the balsamic glaze over the chicken and top with toasted pine nuts.

Exchanges

1/2 Carbohydrate
4 Very Lean Meat
1 1/2 Fat

Calories 231
  Calories from Fat . . . 94
Total Fat . . . . 10 g
  Saturated Fat . . . . . 2.1 g
Cholesterol . . . . 69 mg
Sodium . . . . 195 mg
Total Carbohydrate . . 8 g
  Dietary Fiber . . . . 1 g
  Sugars . . . . 5 g
Protein . . . . 28 g

Chicken Sauté with Lemon and Fennel

4 Servings / Serving Size: 4 oz

4 4-oz boneless, skinless chicken breasts
1/2 tsp salt
1/4 tsp fresh ground black pepper
1 Tbsp olive oil
3 Tbsp dry white wine
2 Tbsp lemon juice
1 tsp grated lemon zest
1 garlic clove, crushed
1/2 tsp fennel seeds

1 Sprinkle the chicken breasts with salt and pepper. Heat the oil in a skillet over medium-high heat. Add the chicken breasts and sauté for a total of 6 minutes.

2 Add the remaining ingredients, cover, reduce the heat to medium low, and cook for about 10 minutes, until the chicken is cooked through. Remove the garlic before serving.

Exchanges
4 Very Lean Meat
1 Fat

Calories	169
Calories from Fat	57
Total Fat	6 g
Saturated Fat	1.3 g
Cholesterol	69 mg
Sodium	352 mg
Total Carbohydrate	1 g
Dietary Fiber	0 g
Sugars	0 g
Protein	25 g

Chicken Scallopini with Sage and Capers

4 Servings / Serving Size: 4 oz

1/4 cup dry white wine
1/3 cup low-fat, reduced-sodium chicken broth
2 tsp capers
3/4 tsp sage
3 Tbsp flour
Salt and pepper (optional)

4 4-oz boneless, skinless chicken breasts, pounded to 1/4-inch thickness
2 Tbsp olive oil, divided
1 tsp arrowroot or cornstarch
2 tsp cold water
1 tsp cold butter, cut into small pieces
2 Tbsp chopped parsley

1 In a small bowl, combine the wine, broth, and capers.

2 Combine the sage, flour, and salt and pepper (if desired) on a plate. Dredge each piece of chicken into the flour mixture and shake off excess.

3 Heat half of the olive oil in a large skillet over medium-high heat. Add two of the chicken breasts and cook on each side for 4–5 minutes. Remove to a platter. Add the remaining oil to the pan and repeat with the other two chicken breasts.

4 Combine the arrowroot or cornstarch and water. Pour the caper mixture into the skillet and heat over medium heat. Bring to a simmer and add the arrowroot/cornstarch mixture. Cook while whisking continuously for about 15 seconds. Whisk in the butter and spoon the sauce over the chicken. Sprinkle with parsley.

Exchanges
1/2 Starch
3 Very Lean Meat
2 Fat

Calories 235	
Calories from Fat. . . 96	
Total Fat . . . . 11 g	
Saturated Fat . . . . . 2.3 g	
Cholesterol . . . . 71 mg	
Sodium . . . . 152 mg	
Total Carbohydrate . . 6 g	
Dietary Fiber . . . . 0 g	
Sugars . . . . 0 g	
Protein . . . . 26 g	

Chicken with Artichokes

4 Servings / Serving Size: 4 oz

4 4-oz boneless, skinless chicken breasts
1/4 tsp salt
1/4 tsp fresh ground black pepper
2 tsp olive oil
1/2 cup dry white wine
1/4 cup low-fat, reduced-sodium chicken broth

2 tsp Dijon mustard
1 tsp cornstarch
1 15-oz can artichokes, drained, rinsed, and halved
2 Tbsp sliced black olives
2 Tbsp minced parsley

1 Sprinkle the chicken with salt and pepper. Heat the oil in large skillet over medium-high heat. Add the chicken and sauté on both sides for a total of 10 minutes. Remove the chicken from the skillet and keep it warm.

2 Mix together the wine, broth, Dijon mustard, and cornstarch and add them to the skillet, scraping up browned bits. Stir the sauce until slightly thickened. Add the artichokes and olives and cook for 1 minute. Add the parsley. Serve the sauce over the chicken.

Exchanges
1 Vegetable
4 Very Lean Meat
1 Fat

Calories 202
  Calories from Fat . . . 53
Total Fat . . . . 6 g
  Saturated Fat . . . . . 1.2 g
Cholesterol . . . . 69 mg
Sodium . . . . 522 mg
Total Carbohydrate . . 6 g
  Dietary Fiber . . . . 1 g
  Sugars . . . . 1 g
Protein . . . . 27 g

Chicken with Fresh Herbs and Shallots

4 Servings / Serving Size: 4 oz

2 tsp olive oil
1 lb boneless, skinless chicken breasts
Salt and pepper to taste
2 garlic cloves, minced
2 shallots, finely minced

3 tomatoes, seeded and diced
1 Tbsp balsamic vinegar
1 Tbsp minced fresh basil
1 Tbsp minced fresh parsley
2 tsp minced fresh oregano
1 tsp minced fresh sage

1 Heat the oil in a large skillet over medium-high heat. Season the chicken breasts with salt and pepper. Sauté the chicken breasts for 3 minutes per side. Remove from the skillet.

2 Add the garlic and shallots to the pan and sauté for 3 minutes. Add the tomatoes and cook for 3 minutes. Add the vinegar and cook for 1 minute. Add the basil, parsley, oregano, and sage and cook for 2 minutes. Put the chicken back in the skillet, cover, and cook for 3 minutes more.

Exchanges
2 Vegetable
3 Very Lean Meat
1 Fat

Calories 188
 Calories from Fat . . . 50
Total Fat . . . . 6 g
 Saturated Fat . . . . . 1.1 g
Cholesterol . . . . 69 mg
Sodium . . . . 71 mg
Total Carbohydrate . . 8 g
 Dietary Fiber . . . . 2 g
 Sugars . . . . 4 g
Protein . . . . 26 g

Chicken with Garlic Spinach

4 Servings / Serving Size: 4 oz

4   4-oz boneless, skinless
chicken breasts
Salt and pepper to taste
3   tsp olive oil, divided
1/2   cup dry Marsala wine
1/3   cup low-fat, reduced-sodium
chicken broth

1 1/2   tsp cornstarch
4   garlic cloves, sliced
1   lb ready-to-eat fresh spinach
leaves

1   Sprinkle the chicken breasts with salt and pepper. Heat half of the oil in a large nonstick skillet over medium-high heat. Add the chicken breasts and sauté on both sides for a total of 10 minutes. Remove the chicken from the skillet.

2   Combine the Marsala, broth, and cornstarch in a measuring cup. Add them to the pan and cook until slightly thickened. Put the chicken back in the pan, cook it for 2 minutes, and then remove it from the pan again.

3   Wipe the pan clean. Add the remaining oil to the pan. Add the garlic and sauté for 20 seconds. Add the spinach and cook for 3 minutes until wilted.

4   To serve, place a mound of the spinach on a plate and add the chicken and the sauce on top.

Exchanges
1/2 Carbohydrate
4 Very Lean Meat
1 Fat

Calories 233
  Calories from Fat . . . 60
Total Fat . . . . 7 g
  Saturated Fat . . . . . 1.3 g
Cholesterol . . . . 69 mg
Sodium . . . . 195 mg
Total Carbohydrate . . 9 g
  Dietary Fiber . . . . 3 g
  Sugars . . . . 4 g
Protein . . . . 29 g

Chicken with Italian Tomatoes and Artichokes

4 Servings / Serving Size: 4 oz

4 4-oz boneless, skinless
   chicken breasts
   Salt and pepper to taste
2 tsp olive oil
2 garlic cloves, minced
1 small onion, diced

1 15-oz can Italian-style diced
   tomatoes, drained slightly
1 1/2 Tbsp prepared pesto sauce
1 15-oz can artichoke hearts,
   drained and halved

1 Season the chicken breasts with salt and pepper. Heat the olive oil in a large nonstick skillet. Add the chicken and sear for 3–4 minutes per side. Remove from the skillet.

2 Add the garlic and onion and sauté for 2 minutes. Add the tomatoes and pesto and simmer for 1 minute. Put the chicken back in the skillet and simmer for 3–4 minutes. Add the artichoke hearts and simmer for 2 minutes.

Exchanges
3 Vegetable
3 Very Lean Meat
1 1/2 Fat

Calories 245
   Calories from Fat . . . 63
Total Fat . . . . 7 g
   Saturated Fat . . . . . 1.4 g
Cholesterol . . . . 69 mg
Sodium . . . . 842 mg
Total Carbohydrate . 17 g
   Dietary Fiber . . . . 2 g
   Sugars . . . . 9 g
Protein . . . . 29 g

Chicken with Peppers I

4 Servings / Serving Size: 4 oz

1 lb boneless, skinless chicken breasts or thighs
Salt and pepper to taste
1 Tbsp olive oil, divided
3 garlic cloves
1 small onion, chopped
1 small red pepper, sliced into thin strips

1 small yellow pepper, sliced into thin strips
1 15-oz can diced tomatoes, drained
2 tsp capers
2 Tbsp freshly grated Parmesan cheese

1 Sprinkle the chicken with salt and pepper. Heat half of the olive oil over medium heat in a large nonstick skillet. Add the chicken and sauté on both sides for a total of 10 minutes. Remove it from the skillet.

2 Add the remaining oil. Add the garlic and onions and sauté for 3 minutes. Add the peppers and sauté for 4 minutes. Add in the drained tomatoes and capers and bring to a boil. Lower the heat and simmer for 3 minutes.

3 Return the chicken to the skillet and sprinkle it with the cheese. Cover and cook for 1 minute until the cheese is slightly melted.

Exchanges

2 Vegetable
3 Very Lean Meat
1 Fat

Calories	213
Calories from Fat	67
Total Fat	7 g
Saturated Fat	1.8 g
Cholesterol	71 mg
Sodium	250 mg
Total Carbohydrate	9 g
Dietary Fiber	2 g
Sugars	6 g
Protein	28 g

Chicken with Peppers II

4 Servings / Serving Size: 4 oz

1 Tbsp olive oil
1 lb boneless, skinless chicken breasts
Salt and pepper to taste
2 Tbsp all-purpose flour
2 Tbsp dry white wine
1 medium onion, chopped
2 garlic cloves, minced
1 small red pepper, seeded and sliced thin

1 small yellow pepper, seeded and sliced thin
1 15-oz can diced no-salt-added tomatoes
2 tsp tomato paste
1 Tbsp minced parsley
3 Tbsp freshly grated Parmesan cheese

1 Heat the oil in a large nonstick skillet over medium-high heat. Sprinkle the chicken with salt and pepper. Dredge each piece in flour. Add the chicken breasts to the skillet, in two batches if necessary. Sauté the chicken on each side for 5 minutes. Remove from the skillet.

2 Add the wine to the skillet, scraping up any browned bits. Add the onion and garlic and sauté for 3 minutes. Add the peppers and sauté for 2 minutes. Add the tomatoes and tomato paste and bring to a boil. Lower the heat and simmer for 5 minutes. Add the parsley.

3 Put the chicken back in the pan, nestling it in the sauce. Cook for 2 minutes. Sprinkle with parsley and Parmesan cheese.

Exchanges
3 Vegetable
3 Lean Meat

Calories 252
  Calories from Fat . . . 72
Total Fat . . . . 8 g
  Saturated Fat . . . . . 2.0 g
Cholesterol . . . . 72 mg
Sodium . . . . 141 mg
Total Carbohydrate . 16 g
  Dietary Fiber . . . . 3 g
  Sugars . . . . 8 g
Protein . . . . 29 g

Chicken with Porcini Mushrooms

4 Servings / Serving Size: 4 oz

Boiling water
1 oz dried porcini mushrooms
1 Tbsp olive oil
1 lb boneless, skinless chicken
   thighs
Salt and pepper to taste

1 medium onion, chopped
2 garlic cloves, minced
1/2 cup dry white wine
2 Tbsp tomato paste

1 In a small heat-proof bowl, pour boiling water over the porcini
mushrooms so that it just covers them. Set aside to soak for
10 minutes.

2 Meanwhile, heat the olive oil in a large nonstick skillet over
medium-high heat. Sprinkle the chicken with salt and pepper and
add half of the chicken thighs. Cook each thigh for 5–6 minutes per side.
Remove and repeat with the remaining chicken thighs.

3 Remove the last batch of
chicken from the skillet. Add
the onion and garlic and sauté for
3 minutes. Drain the mushrooms,
reserving the liquid.

4 Combine the wine and tomato
paste. Add to the skillet. Add
the mushrooms and the mushroom
liquid. Return the chicken thighs to
the skillet, cover, and simmer for
8 minutes. Serve the chicken with
the mushroom sauce spooned on
top.

Exchanges
2 Vegetable
3 Lean Meat
1 Fat

Calories 266
  Calories from Fat . . 116
Total Fat . . . . 13 g
  Saturated Fat . . . . . 3.1 g
Cholesterol . . . . 81 mg
Sodium . . . . 84 mg
Total Carbohydrate . 11 g
  Dietary Fiber . . . . 2 g
  Sugars . . . . 5 g
Protein . . . . 24 g

Chicken with Portobello Mushroom Sauce

4 Servings / Serving Size: 4 oz

4 4-oz boneless, skinless chicken breasts
Salt and pepper to taste
2 tsp olive oil
1/2 small onion, diced
2 garlic cloves, minced
1 large portobello mushroom cleaned, stemmed, and diced into 1/2-inch pieces

1 tsp minced fresh rosemary (1/2 tsp dried)
1/2 tsp dried thyme
1/4 cup flour
1 15-oz can low-fat, reduced-sodium chicken broth
1 Tbsp minced parsley

1 Sprinkle the chicken with salt and pepper to taste. Heat the oil in a large nonstick skillet over medium-high heat. Add the chicken in batches if necessary and sauté for 4 minutes per side. Remove from the skillet.

2 Add the onion and garlic and sauté for 3 minutes. Add the mushroom and sauté until it browns and begins to release its juices. Add the rosemary, thyme, and flour, coating the vegetables well with the flour.

3 Add the broth and bring to a boil. Lower the heat and put the chicken back in the skillet. Cover and cook over low heat for 5 minutes until the chicken is cooked through. Sprinkle with parsley.

Exchanges
1/2 Starch
4 Very Lean Meat
1/2 Fat

Calories 201
  Calories from Fat . . . 48
Total Fat . . . . 5 g
  Saturated Fat . . . . . 1.1 g
Cholesterol . . . . 69 mg
Sodium . . . . 320 mg
Total Carbohydrate . . 9 g
  Dietary Fiber . . . . 1 g
  Sugars . . . . 2 g
Protein . . . . 28 g

Chicken with Rosemary Sauce

4 Servings / Serving Size: 4 oz

2 tsp olive oil
1 lb boneless, skinless chicken breasts
Salt and pepper to taste
1 garlic clove, minced
2 shallots, minced
1/2 cup low-fat, reduced-sodium chicken broth

2 tsp finely minced fresh rosemary leaves
1/2 tsp Dijon mustard
1 tsp cornstarch
1 Tbsp water
2 tsp fresh lemon juice

1 Heat the oil in a large skillet over medium-high heat. Sprinkle the chicken with the salt and pepper. Sauté the chicken breasts for 4 minutes per side. Remove from the skillet and set aside. Add the garlic and shallots and sauté for 2 minutes.

2 Mix together the broth, rosemary, and mustard. Add them to the skillet and bring to a boil. Lower the heat and simmer the sauce for 3 minutes. Mix the cornstarch and water together, add them to the skillet, and stir until the mixture is slightly thickened.

3 Put the chicken back in the skillet and add the lemon juice. Simmer the chicken for 2 minutes more.

Exchanges
4 Very Lean Meat
1/2 Fat

Calories 167
 Calories from Fat . . . 47
Total Fat . . . . 5 g
 Saturated Fat . . . . . 1.1 g
Cholesterol . . . . 69 mg
Sodium . . . . 139 mg
Total Carbohydrate . . 3 g
 Dietary Fiber . . . . 0 g
 Sugars . . . . 1 g
Protein . . . . 26 g

Chicken with Sage and Lemon

4 Servings / Serving Size: 4 oz

2 Tbsp flour
Salt and pepper to taste
Pinch crushed red pepper
1 lb boneless, skinless chicken
  cutlets
1 Tbsp olive oil, divided
2 garlic cloves, minced

2 tsp fresh chopped sage
1/4 cup dry white wine
3/4 cup low-fat, reduced-sodium
  chicken broth
2 tsp fresh lemon juice
1/2 tsp butter

1 Mix the flour, salt, pepper, and crushed red pepper on a plate. Dredge the chicken in the flour mixture. Heat half of the olive oil in a large nonstick skillet over medium-high heat. Add the chicken and sauté, in batches if necessary, for 4–5 minutes per side. Remove the chicken from the skillet.

2 Add the remaining olive oil to the pan. Add the garlic and sage and sauté for 30 seconds. Add the white wine, broth, and lemon juice and bring to a boil. Lower the heat and reduce for 1–2 minutes. Swirl in the butter. Pour the sauce over the chicken.

Exchanges
4 Very Lean Meat
1 Fat

Calories 193
  Calories from Fat . . . 61
Total Fat . . . . 7 g
  Saturated Fat . . . . . 1.6 g
Cholesterol . . . . 70 mg
Sodium . . . . 158 mg
Total Carbohydrate . . 4 g
  Dietary Fiber . . . . 0 g
  Sugars . . . . 1 g
Protein . . . . 26 g

Chicken with Shallot Sauce

4 Servings / Serving Size: 4 oz

4 4-oz chicken cutlets (about 1/4 inch thick)

4 oz minced extra lean, low-sodium ham

1 oz freshly grated Parmesan cheese

1 tsp dried oregano
Pepper to taste

1 1/2 Tbsp olive oil, divided

1/2 tsp butter

2 small shallots, minced

1/3 cup dry white wine

2 tsp lemon juice

1 tsp minced fresh rosemary (1/2 tsp dried)

1 Preheat the oven to 350 degrees. Lay the four chicken cutlets on a work surface.

2 In a bowl, combine the ham, cheese, oregano, and pepper. Place 1/4 of the ham mixture in the center of each cutlet and then roll the chicken up tightly.

3 Heat 1 Tbsp of the oil in a large nonstick skillet. Add the chicken, seam side down, and sauté for 4–5 minutes per side.

4 Remove the chicken from the skillet and place it on a baking sheet. Bake it in the oven until it is cooked through, about 7–8 minutes.

5 Meanwhile, add the remaining oil and the butter to the skillet and cook over medium heat until the butter melts. Add the shallots and sauté for 2 minutes. Add the white wine and lemon juice, bring to a boil, lower the heat, and cook for 2 minutes. Add the rosemary and cook for 1 minute.

6 Remove the chicken from the oven and pour the shallot sauce over it.

Exchanges
4 Very Lean Meat
2 Fat

Calories 235
  Calories from Fat . . . 85
Total Fat . . . . 9 g
  Saturated Fat . . . . . 2.3 g
Cholesterol . . . . 84 mg
Sodium . . . . 307 mg
Total Carbohydrate . . 3 g
  Dietary Fiber . . . . 1 g
  Sugars . . . . 2 g
Protein . . . . 31 g

Easy Mediterranean-Style Chicken Salad

4 Servings / Serving Size: 1 cup

8 oz precooked chicken strips (such as Perdue)
1 15-oz can water-packed artichoke hearts, drained and halved
1 7-oz jar roasted red peppers, sliced
1 cup halved cherry tomatoes
2 Tbsp black olives
   Juice of 1 lemon
2 Tbsp red wine vinegar
1 1/2 Tbsp olive oil
1 Tbsp minced chives

Combine all ingredients, cover, and refrigerate a half hour before serving.

Exchanges
2 Vegetable
2 Very Lean Meat
1 Fat

Calories	154
Calories from Fat	62
Total Fat	7 g
Saturated Fat	1.0 g
Cholesterol	34 mg
Sodium	534 mg
Total Carbohydrate	11 g
Dietary Fiber	2 g
Sugars	4 g
Protein	14 g

Herb Grilled Chicken with Walnut Pesto

4 Servings / Serving Size: 4 oz

1/4 cup minced basil

2 sprigs fresh rosemary, chopped

6 sprigs fresh thyme, chopped

1/4 cup walnuts

3 cloves garlic, minced

3 Tbsp fat-free, reduced-sodium chicken broth

1 Tbsp plus 2 tsp olive oil
Salt and pepper to taste

2 Tbsp freshly grated Parmesan cheese

4 4-oz boneless chicken breasts, skins on, 1 inch thick

1 In a food processor, add the herbs and pulse until fine. Add the walnuts, garlic, broth, and 1 Tbsp of olive oil and pulse until the mixture is incorporated but still slightly chunky. Remove to a bowl and add the salt, pepper, and cheese.

2 Cut a pocket into each chicken breast. Stuff some of the pesto mixture into the pocket and rub some under the skin.

3 Rub each chicken breast with the remaining olive oil. Grill or broil the chicken for 5–8 minutes per side, turning frequently. Remove skin before eating.

Exchanges
4 Very Lean Meat
2 Fat

Calories 239
  Calories from Fat. . 127
Total Fat . . . . 14 g
  Saturated Fat . . . . . 2.5 g
Cholesterol . . . . 65 mg
Sodium . . . . 100 mg
Total Carbohydrate . . 2 g
  Dietary Fiber . . . . 1 g
  Sugars . . . . 1 g
Protein . . . . 25 g

Italian Chicken Salad with Walnuts

4 Servings / Serving Size: 1 cup

1 lb boneless, skinless chicken breasts	**10** pitted Kalamata olives
Water	**2** Tbsp minced parsley
4 peppercorns	
1/2 Tbsp olive oil	**DRESSING**
1/2 cup walnuts	**1** Tbsp olive oil
1 medium red pepper, diced	**1** Tbsp fresh lemon juice
1 tsp dried oregano	**1** Tbsp red wine vinegar
1/2 tsp dried basil	**1** garlic clove, minced
1 15-oz can artichoke hearts, drained and halved	**1/2** tsp sugar
	1/2 tsp salt
	1/4 tsp black pepper

1 Place the chicken breasts in a large skillet with enough water to cover them. Add the peppercorns. Bring to a boil over high heat, lower the heat, cover, and simmer for 7–10 minutes or until cooked through. Remove the chicken from the skillet with a slotted spoon, place on a plate, and refrigerate.

2 Heat the oil in a skillet over medium heat. Add the walnuts and sauté for 2 minutes. Add the red pepper, oregano, and basil and sauté for 3 minutes. Remove from the heat and let cool.

3 Meanwhile, in a salad bowl, combine the artichoke hearts, olives, and parsley.

4 Combine all dressing ingredients. Add the walnut mixture to the salad. Cut the chicken into 1-inch cubes and add it to the salad. Pour the dressing over it. Toss well and serve.

Exchanges

2 Vegetable
4 Very Lean Meat
3 Fat

Calories 333	
Calories from Fat . 173	
Total Fat . . . . 19 g	
Saturated Fat . . . . 2.6 g	
Cholesterol . . . . 70 mg	
Sodium . . . . 635 mg	
Total Carbohydrate . 11 g	
Dietary Fiber . . . . . . 3 g	
Sugars . . . . 4 g	
Protein . . . . 31 g	

Rosemary Lemon Chicken Thighs

4 Servings / Serving Size: 4 oz

2 Tbsp fresh lemon juice
1 Tbsp olive oil
1/2 small onion, minced
2 garlic cloves, minced
2 tsp fresh minced rosemary (1 tsp dried)
Salt and pepper to taste
1 lb boneless, skinless chicken thighs
Nonstick cooking spray

1 Preheat an oven broiler. In a large bowl, combine all ingredients. Let the chicken marinate for 10 minutes.

2 Place the chicken thighs on a broiler pan sprayed with cooking spray. Broil the chicken for 6–7 minutes per side until cooked through.

Exchanges
3 Lean Meat
1/2 Fat

Calories 205
  Calories from Fat . . 104
Total Fat . . . . 12 g
  Saturated Fat . . . . . 2.9 g
Cholesterol . . . . 81 mg
Sodium . . . . 77 mg
Total Carbohydrate . . 1 g
  Dietary Fiber . . . . . . 0 g
  Sugars . . . . 1 g
Protein . . . . 22 g

Rosemary Olive Chicken

4 Servings / Serving Size: 4 oz

1 lb boneless, skinless chicken thighs
2 Tbsp flour
2 tsp dried rosemary
   Salt and pepper to taste
2 tsp olive oil
1 onion, chopped
2 garlic cloves, minced
2/3 cup low-fat, reduced-sodium chicken broth

1/4 cup dry white wine
2 tsp lemon juice
1 tsp cornstarch
1 Tbsp water
2 Tbsp pitted, sliced Kalamata olives
2 Tbsp minced parsley

1 Coat each chicken thigh with flour that has been mixed with the rosemary, salt, and pepper. Shake off excess. Heat the oil in a large nonstick skillet. Sauté the chicken thighs, in batches if necessary, until browned on both sides, about 4–5 minutes per side. Remove from the skillet.

2 Add the onion and garlic to the pan and sauté for 4 minutes. Combine the broth, wine, and lemon juice and add them to the pan. Bring to a boil, and then lower the heat. Combine the cornstarch and water and add to the pan. Cook until the sauce thickens slightly.

3 Return the chicken and any accumulated juices to the pan, cover, and simmer for 2 minutes. Add the olives and parsley to the pan and cook for 1 minute.

Exchanges
1/2 Starch
3 Lean Meat

Calories	202
Calories from Fat	87
Total Fat	10 g
Saturated Fat	2.3 g
Cholesterol	62 mg
Sodium	176 mg
Total Carbohydrate	9 g
Dietary Fiber	1 g
Sugars	3 g
Protein	19 g

Beef (Manzo)

Filet with Portobello Mushrooms

4 Servings / Serving Size: 4–5 oz

Nonstick cooking spray
4 4–5-oz filet mignons
Salt and pepper to taste
1 tsp olive oil
1 garlic clove, minced
1 small onion, halved and thinly sliced

1 large portobello mushroom, stemmed, cleaned, and thinly sliced
1/2 cup low-fat, reduced-sodium chicken broth
2 tsp minced fresh basil

1 Spray a large skillet with cooking spray. Heat the pan over medium-high heat. Season each filet with salt and pepper. Place the filets in the skillet and cook for 4 minutes per side. Remove the filets from the skillet and place them on a baking sheet. Either cover the filets and keep them warm or continue to roast them in a 400-degree oven until done as desired.

2 Meanwhile, add the olive oil to the skillet. Add the garlic and onion and sauté for 4 minutes. Add the portobello mushroom slices and continue to cook until they soften and brown, about 5 minutes. Add the chicken broth and bring to a boil. Lower the heat and simmer for 2–3 minutes. Add the basil.

3 Serve the filets topped with the portobello mushrooms mixture.

Exchanges
3 Lean Meat

Calories	176
Calories from Fat	74
Total Fat	8 g
Saturated Fat	2.9 g
Cholesterol	60 mg
Sodium	109 mg
Total Carbohydrate	3 g
Dietary Fiber	1 g
Sugars	2 g
Protein	21 g

Garlic-Infused Beef Kebabs

4 Servings / Serving Size: 4 oz

1 lb lean beef sirloin, cut into 1 1/2-inch pieces
   Salt and pepper to taste
12 cherry tomatoes
2 Tbsp olive oil
4 garlic cloves, finely minced
1 Tbsp minced fresh rosemary

1 Season the beef with salt and pepper.

2 Thread the beef cubes and cherry tomatoes evenly onto 4 metal skewers.

3 Combine the olive oil, garlic, and rosemary. Brush the kebabs with the garlic and oil mixture.

4 Prepare a hot grill or an oven broiler. Grill or broil the kebabs for 4–5 minutes per side, turning once. Baste with any remaining garlic and oil mixture.

Exchanges
3 Lean Meat

Calories	175
Calories from Fat	67
Total Fat	7 g
Saturated Fat	2.2 g
Cholesterol	65 mg
Sodium	54 mg
Total Carbohydrate	3 g
Dietary Fiber	1 g
Sugars	2 g
Protein	23 g

Sirloin Steak with Rosemary

4 Servings / Serving Size: 4 oz

1 lb lean boneless sirloin steak
 Salt and pepper to taste
1 long branch fresh rosemary
1 Tbsp olive oil

1 Heat an outdoor grill to high heat or set an oven broiler to high with the rack 4–6 inches from the heat source.

2 Sprinkle the steak with salt and pepper. Place the steak on the grill or broiler rack. Dip the stem of rosemary into the olive oil. Brush one side of the steak with the olive oil and grill for 5–6 minutes. Turn the steak over and repeat with the olive oil. Grill for another 5–6 minutes until done as desired.

Exchanges
3 Lean Meat

Calories	184
Calories from Fat	74
Total Fat	8 g
Saturated Fat	2.3 g
Cholesterol	49 mg
Sodium	54 mg
Total Carbohydrate	0 g
Dietary Fiber	0 g
Sugars	0 g
Protein	26 g

Steak Milanese

4 Servings / Serving Size: 4 oz

4 4-oz beef cubed steaks
   Salt and pepper to taste
1–2 egg whites
   1 Tbsp water
1/2 cup dry seasoned bread crumbs
   1 Tbsp olive oil
   1 tomato, seeded and chopped
1/4 cup minced parsley

1 Season the steaks with salt and pepper.

2 Combine the egg whites and water in a bowl. Dip each steak into the egg mixture and then coat with the bread crumbs. Repeat with each steak.

3 Heat the oil in a large skillet over medium heat. Add the steaks in two batches and sauté until golden brown, 5–6 minutes for each steak, turning once.

4 Sprinkle each steak with chopped tomato and parsley.

Exchanges
1 Starch
3 Lean Meat

Calories	233
Calories from Fat	81
Total Fat	9 g
Saturated Fat	2.3 g
Cholesterol	64 mg
Sodium	450 mg
Total Carbohydrate	12 g
Dietary Fiber	1 g
Sugars	2 g
Protein	24 g

Steak Pizzaiola

4 Servings / Serving Size: 4 oz

2 tsp olive oil
1 lb flank steak
1 small onion, chopped
3 garlic cloves, minced
1 cup canned plum tomatoes,
   coarsely chopped
1 Tbsp minced fresh oregano
   (1 tsp dried)

2 tsp balsamic vinegar
1/4 cup black olives, pitted and
   halved
1 tsp sugar
   Salt and pepper to taste

1 Heat the olive oil in a large skillet over medium-high heat. Add the flank steak and cook for 5–6 minutes per side for medium rare, longer if desired. Remove the steak from the skillet and keep warm.

2 Add the onion and garlic to the pan drippings and sauté for 3 minutes. Add the tomatoes and oregano and bring to a boil. Lower the heat and simmer for 5 minutes. Add the vinegar and olives and simmer for 3 minutes. Add the sugar and cook for 1 minute. Season with salt and pepper. Serve the steak with the sauce.

Exchanges
1 Vegetable
3 Lean Meat

Calories	208
Calories from Fat	82
Total Fat	9 g
Saturated Fat	2.9 g
Cholesterol	39 mg
Sodium	210 mg
Total Carbohydrate	8 g
Dietary Fiber	1 g
Sugars	5 g
Protein	23 g

Veal Marsala

4 Servings / Serving Size: 4 oz

1 lb veal scallopini	**1/3** cup low-fat, reduced-sodium
4 Tbsp flour, divided	chicken broth
1 Tbsp olive oil	**1/2** cup dry Marsala wine
1/2 Tbsp butter	**1/4** tsp salt
1 cup presliced mushrooms	**1** Tbsp chopped parsley

1 Dredge the veal in 2 Tbsp flour and shake off excess. Heat the oil in a nonstick skillet over medium-high heat. Sauté the veal for about 90 seconds on each side. Remove the meat from the pan and place on a warm platter.

2 Add the rest of the ingredients, except for the remaining 2 Tbsp of flour and the parsley. Bring to a simmer over medium heat. Slowly sift the remaining flour into the sauce until it reaches the desired thickness. You may not need all the flour.

3 Return the meat to the pan, warm it, and cover it with the sauce. Garnish with parsley and serve.

Exchanges
1/2 Carbohydrate
3 Lean Meat
1/2 Fat

Calories 245
 Calories from Fat . . . 75
Total Fat . . . . 8 g
 Saturated Fat . . . . . 2.4 g
Cholesterol . . . . 80 mg
Sodium . . . . 256 mg
Total Carbohydrate . 10 g
 Dietary Fiber . . . . 0 g
 Sugars . . . . 3 g
Protein . . . . 25 g

Veal Scallopini with Olives and Pine Nuts

4 Servings / Serving Size: 4 oz

2 tsp olive oil
1 lb veal scallopini
2 Tbsp flour
Salt and pepper to taste
Nonstick cooking spray
1 cup diced onion
2 garlic cloves, minced

2 medium tomatoes, seeded and chopped
1/2 cup dry white wine
10 black olives, pitted and halved
2 Tbsp pine nuts, toasted
1/2 cup torn basil leaves

1 Heat the oil in a large skillet over medium heat. Dredge the veal in flour mixed with salt and pepper. Add the veal in batches, sautéing for 2–3 minutes per side. Remove from the skillet.

2 Spray the pan with cooking spray, add the onion and garlic to the pan, and sauté for 3 minutes. Add the tomatoes and sauté for 3 minutes. Add the white wine and bring to a boil. Then lower the heat and simmer for 2 minutes. Add the olives and pine nuts and cook for 1 minute. Add the basil and cook for 1 minute. Taste and correct the seasoning. Serve the olive and tomato mixture over the veal.

Exchanges

3 Vegetable
3 Lean Meat
1/2 Fat

Calories	262
Calories from Fat	88
Total Fat	10 g
Saturated Fat	2.0 g
Cholesterol	77 mg
Sodium	164 mg
Total Carbohydrate	13 g
Dietary Fiber	3 g
Sugars	6 g
Protein	27 g

Veal with Leeks and Mushrooms

4 Servings / Serving Size: 4 oz

1 lb veal scallopini
1 1/2 Tbsp flour
Salt and pepper to taste
3 tsp olive oil, divided
2 leeks, bottoms only, washed, halved, and thinly sliced

2 garlic cloves, minced
8 oz sliced cremini mushrooms (or regular button mushrooms)
1/4 cup dry white wine
Juice of 1 small lemon
1/2 tsp lemon zest

1 Coat the veal with flour mixed with salt and pepper. Shake off the excess. Heat 2 tsp of the oil in a large nonstick skillet. Add the veal and cook for 1–2 minutes per side. Remove from the pan.

2 Add the remaining 1 tsp of oil. Add the leeks and garlic and sauté for 4 minutes. Add the mushrooms and sauté for 4 minutes until they begin to release their juices. Remove the veal, leeks, and mushrooms from the skillet.

3 Add the wine to the skillet and cook for 30 seconds. Add the lemon and lemon zest and cook 1 minute. Put the veal, leeks, and mushrooms back in the skillet and heat through.

Exchanges
2 Vegetable
3 Lean Meat

Calories 223
Calories from Fat. . . 64
Total Fat . . . . 7 g
Saturated Fat . . . . . 1.5 g
Cholesterol . . . . 77 mg
Sodium . . . . 69 mg
Total Carbohydrate . 12 g
Dietary Fiber . . . . 2 g
Sugars . . . . 3 g
Protein . . . . 26 g

Veal with Leeks and Zucchini

4 Servings / Serving Size: 4 oz

1 lb veal scallopini
Salt and pepper to taste
1 Tbsp olive oil
1 garlic clove, minced
1 leek, white part only, washed
and diced

1 small zucchini, diced
3 Tbsp white wine
1 tsp dried thyme
1 tsp dried oregano

1 Sprinkle the veal with salt and pepper. Heat the oil in a large skillet over medium-high heat. Add the veal in batches if necessary and sauté for 1–2 minutes per side. Remove from the skillet.

2 Add the garlic and leeks to the skillet and sauté for 4 minutes. Add the zucchini and sauté for 4 minutes and then add the wine. Add the thyme and oregano and sauté for 2 minutes. Put the veal back in the skillet, cover, and cook on low for 2 minutes.

Exchanges
1 Vegetable
3 Lean Meat

Calories	189
Calories from Fat	62
Total Fat	7 g
Saturated Fat	1.5 g
Cholesterol	77 mg
Sodium	64 mg
Total Carbohydrate	5 g
Dietary Fiber	1 g
Sugars	2 g
Protein	25 g

Veal with Sage and Garlic

4 Servings / Serving Size: 4 oz

2 tsp olive oil
1 lb veal scallopini
3 garlic cloves, minced
1/2 cup diced onion
2 Tbsp dry white wine
3/4 cup low-fat, reduced-sodium
   chicken broth

1 Tbsp minced fresh sage
1 tsp capers
1 tsp cornstarch
1 Tbsp water
1 Tbsp fresh minced parsley

1 Heat the oil in a large skillet over medium-high heat. Add the veal scallopini, in batches if necessary. Cook for 1–2 minutes per side. Remove from the skillet and set aside.

2 Add the garlic and onion to the skillet and sauté for 3 minutes. Add the white wine, scraping up any browned bits. Cook the wine for 2 minutes. Add the broth and bring to a boil. Lower the heat and simmer for 2 minutes. Add the sage and cook for 3 minutes. Add the capers.

3 Combine the cornstarch and water and add to the skillet. Cook the sauce over medium heat for 1–2 minutes until slightly thickened. Put the veal back in the skillet and cook it in the sauce for 1–2 minutes. Sprinkle with parsley.

Exchanges
3 Lean Meat

Calories	172
Calories from Fat	51
Total Fat	6 g
Saturated Fat	1.3 g
Cholesterol	77 mg
Sodium	173 mg
Total Carbohydrate	4 g
Dietary Fiber	1 g
Sugars	2 g
Protein	25 g

Pork (Maiale)

Pork Chops with Sage and Rosemary

4 Servings / Serving Size: 4 oz

2 tsp olive oil
4 4-oz boneless pork loin chops
1 Tbsp flour
Salt and pepper to taste
1 Tbsp minced fresh rosemary
2 tsp minced fresh sage
1/2 cup dry white wine
1 cup low-fat, reduced-sodium chicken broth

1 Heat the olive oil in a large skillet over medium-high heat. Dredge the pork chops in flour mixed with salt and pepper. Sauté the pork chops in the oil for 3 minutes per side.

2 Add the herbs and cook for 2 minutes. Add the wine and bring to a boil, letting the wine evaporate. Add the broth, cover, and simmer for 7 minutes.

3 Remove the pork from the skillet. Raise the heat and reduce the pan juice by half. Serve the pan juice over the pork.

Exchanges
3 Lean Meat
1/2 Fat

Calories 195
  Calories from Fat . . . 85
Total Fat . . . . 9 g
  Saturated Fat . . . . . 2.9 g
Cholesterol . . . . 58 mg
Sodium . . . . 172 mg
Total Carbohydrate . . 2 g
  Dietary Fiber . . . . 0 g
  Sugars . . . . 0 g
Protein . . . . 22 g

Pork Cutlets with Bacon and Onions

4 Servings / Serving Size: 4 oz

2 slices lean bacon
1 large onion, cut in half and sliced
2 tsp balsamic vinegar
Nonstick cooking spray

4 4-oz pork cutlets, trimmed of excess fat
1/2 tsp salt
1/4 tsp fresh ground black pepper

1 Cook the bacon in a large nonstick skillet for about 6 minutes. Remove the bacon from the skillet and chop it into bite-sized pieces.

2 Drain all but 1 tsp of the fat. Add the onion to the skillet and cook for 7–8 minutes. Add the balsamic vinegar and cook for 1 minute. Remove the onions from the skillet. Add the bacon to the onions and keep warm.

3 Wipe the skillet clean and spray with cooking spray. Sprinkle the pork with salt and pepper. Sauté the pork over medium heat for 4–5 minutes per side. Serve the bacon and onion mixture over the pork.

Exchanges
1 Vegetable
3 Lean Meat

Calories	188
Calories from Fat	61
Total Fat	7 g
Saturated Fat	2.3 g
Cholesterol	69 mg
Sodium	391 mg
Total Carbohydrate	6 g
Dietary Fiber	1 g
Sugars	4 g
Protein	25 g

Pork Loin Chops with Herbed Mustard Sauce

4 Servings / Serving Size: 4–5 oz

4 pork loin chops
(4–5 oz each)
Salt and pepper to taste
2 Tbsp all-purpose flour
1 1/2 Tbsp olive oil
1/2 onion, chopped
4 garlic cloves, thickly
sliced

1 Tbsp minced fresh thyme
1 Tbsp minced fresh rosemary
1/4 cup dry white wine
1/2 cup low-fat, reduced-sodium
chicken broth
2 Tbsp Dijon mustard

1 Sprinkle both sides of each pork loin chop with salt and pepper. Dredge each piece in the flour. In a large skillet, heat the oil over medium heat. Add the pork and cook for 4 minutes per side. Remove from the skillet.

2 Add the onion, garlic, and herbs and sauté for 3 minutes. Add the wine and bring to a boil. Cook for 1 minute. Add the chicken broth and bring to a boil. Add the mustard.

3 Put the pork back in the skillet with any accumulated juices. Cook for 1 minute. Serve the pork with the sauce spooned on top.

Exchanges
1/2 Starch
3 Lean Meat

Calories 199
  Calories from Fat. . . 90
Total Fat . . . . 10 g
  Saturated Fat . . . . . 2.4 g
Cholesterol . . . . 47 mg
Sodium . . . . 279 mg
Total Carbohydrate . . 7 g
  Dietary Fiber . . . . 1 g
  Sugars . . . . 3 g
Protein . . . . 18 g

Pork Medallions with Pine Nuts and White Wine

4 Servings / Serving Size: 4 oz

4 4-oz pork medallions,
   trimmed of fat
1 Tbsp flour
1 tsp butter
1 tsp olive oil

2 Tbsp minced chives
1/3 cup dry white wine
1/4 tsp salt
1/4 tsp fresh ground black pepper
1 1/2 Tbsp pine nuts

1 Dredge the pork in the flour and shake off excess. Heat the butter and oil in a large skillet over medium-high heat. Add the pork and sauté on both sides for a total of 5 minutes.

2 Add the chives and wine, lower the heat, cover, and cook for about 5 minutes. Season with salt and pepper.

3 Meanwhile, lightly toast the pine nuts in a dry skillet over medium heat, about 3–4 minutes. Add the pine nuts to the pork and serve.

Exchanges
3 Lean Meat
1/2 Fat

Calories 192
  Calories from Fat . . . 72
Total Fat . . . . 8 g
  Saturated Fat . . . . . 2.5 g
Cholesterol . . . . 68 mg
Sodium . . . . 200 mg
Total Carbohydrate . . 2 g
  Dietary Fiber . . . . 0 g
  Sugars . . . . 0 g
Protein . . . . 25 g

Pork Oreganata

4 Servings / Serving Size: 4 oz

4 4-oz boneless pork loin chops
1 Tbsp flour
Salt and pepper to taste
1 Tbsp olive oil, divided
3 Tbsp dry white wine or reduced-sodium, low-fat chicken broth

4 garlic cloves, minced
2 Tbsp fresh oregano, chopped
1/4 tsp dried thyme

1 Coat the pork chops with flour that has been mixed with salt and pepper. Heat half of the olive oil in a large nonstick pan over medium-high heat. Add the pork chops and sauté for 3–4 minutes per side. Remove from the skillet.

2 Add the white wine or broth and boil for 1 minute. Add the remaining olive oil and the garlic and sauté for 2 minutes. Add the oregano and thyme and cook for 1 minute.

3 Put the pork chops back in the pan and coat them with the garlic and oregano.

Exchanges
3 Lean Meat
1/2 Fat

Calories 204
  Calories from Fat. . . 96
Total Fat . . . . 11 g
  Saturated Fat . . . . . 3.0 g
Cholesterol . . . . 58 mg
Sodium . . . . 48 mg
Total Carbohydrate . . 3 g
  Dietary Fiber . . . . 1 g
  Sugars . . . . 1 g
Protein . . . . 22 g

Pork Salad with Pine Nuts and Basil

4 Servings / Serving Size: 4 oz

1 lb lean boneless pork loin chops
Nonstick cooking spray
Salt and pepper to taste
1 Tbsp toasted pine nuts

SALAD

1 medium red pepper, sliced thin
1 medium yellow pepper, sliced thin

1/2 red onion, sliced thin
4 plum tomatoes, cut into 1/2-inch chunks
1/4 cup chopped fresh basil
3 Tbsp balsamic vinegar
1 1/2 Tbsp olive oil
4 cups torn salad greens of choice

1 Preheat the oven broiler. Place the pork loin chops on a broiler pan sprayed with cooking spray. Season with salt and pepper. Place the pork chops 4–6 inches from the heat source and broil for 4 minutes per side. Remove from the heat and set aside.

2 Combine the ingredients for the salad, except for the salad greens.

3 Slice the pork into thin strips. Line a platter with the salad greens. Pile the other salad ingredients on top of the greens. Top with the sliced pork. Garnish with the pine nuts.

Exchanges
2 Vegetable
3 Lean Meat
1 Fat

Calories	266
Calories from Fat	126
Total Fat	14 g
Saturated Fat	3.5 g
Cholesterol	58 mg
Sodium	61 mg
Total Carbohydrate	13 g
Dietary Fiber	3 g
Sugars	7 g
Protein	24 g

Rosemary Pork Chops

4 Servings / Serving Size: 4 oz

- **1** Tbsp olive oil
- **1 1/2** tsp rosemary, crushed
- **2** tsp bottled minced garlic
- **1/2** tsp salt
- **1/4** tsp black pepper
- **4** 4-oz boneless pork loin chops

1 Preheat the oven broiler. In a small bowl, combine all the ingredients except the pork chops. Rub the mixture over the pork chops.

2 Place the pork chops on a broiler pan and broil for 6–8 minutes, turning once, until the meat is cooked through.

Exchanges
3 Lean Meat
1/2 Fat

Calories	187
Calories from Fat	95
Total Fat	11 g
Saturated Fat	3.0 g
Cholesterol	58 mg
Sodium	338 mg
Total Carbohydrate	1 g
Dietary Fiber	0 g
Sugars	0 g
Protein	21 g

Sautéed Pork with Lemon and Parsley

4 Servings / Serving Size: 4 oz

4 Tbsp dry bread crumbs
1/2 tsp dried basil
1/2 tsp dried thyme
1/2 tsp dried oregano
4 4-oz boneless pork loin chops
2 tsp olive oil

1/4 cup chopped onion
1 garlic clove, minced
1 cup low-fat, reduced-sodium chicken broth
1 Tbsp lemon juice
1 tsp capers
Salt and pepper to taste

1 Combine the bread crumbs, basil, thyme, and oregano on a flat plate. Dredge the pork in the bread crumb mixture, coating both sides.

2 Heat the oil in a large skillet over medium-high heat. Add the pork and sauté for 3–4 minutes per side. Remove from the pan. Add the onion and garlic to the pan and sauté for 3 minutes.

3 Add the broth and lemon juice to the skillet and bring to a boil. Reduce the liquid by half. Add the capers, salt, and pepper. Put the pork back in the skillet and simmer for 1–2 minutes.

Exchanges
1/2 Starch
2 Lean Meat
1/2 Fat

Calories 166
 Calories from Fat . . . 70
Total Fat . . . . 8 g
 Saturated Fat . . . . . 2.1 g
Cholesterol . . . . 41 mg
Sodium . . . . 238 mg
Total Carbohydrate . . 7 g
 Dietary Fiber . . . . 1 g
 Sugars . . . . 1 g
Protein . . . . 17 g

Lamb (Agnello)

Lamb Chops with Olives

4 Servings / Serving Size: 4 oz

- **4** 4-oz lean lamb chops
  Salt and pepper to taste
- **2** tsp dried oregano
- **1 1/2** Tbsp olive oil
- **1/3** cup dry white wine
- **5** small pitted Kalamata olives, chopped
- **2** Tbsp balsamic vinegar

1 Sprinkle the lamb with salt, pepper, and oregano. Heat the oil in a large skillet over medium heat. Add the lamb chops and cook for about 4 minutes per side. Remove the lamb from the skillet.

2 Add the white wine to the skillet, scraping up browned bits. Add the olives and vinegar and bring to a boil. Lower the heat and simmer until the liquid is reduced by half.

3 Drizzle the olive and vinegar sauce over the lamb.

Exchanges
2 Lean Meat
1 Fat

Calories	167
Calories from Fat	92
Total Fat	10 g
Saturated Fat	2.4 g
Cholesterol	46 mg
Sodium	76 mg
Total Carbohydrate	2 g
Dietary Fiber	0 g
Sugars	1 g
Protein	15 g

Spiedino of Lamb

4 Servings / Serving Size: 4 oz

1 lb lean lamb shoulder, boneless, cut into 1-inch cubes
Salt and pepper to taste
4 very long rosemary sprigs or 8 wooden skewers that have been soaked in warm water for 1 hour
2 Tbsp olive oil

1 Preheat an outdoor grill to medium high or an oven broiler with the rack set 6 inches below the heat source. Toss the lamb cubes with salt and pepper.

2 Thread the lamb cubes onto all four rosemary sprigs or onto four sets of two wooden skewers placed side by side.

3 Place the sprigs or skewers on the rack or broiler pan and brush with olive oil. Grill or broil the lamb for about 4 minutes per side.

Exchanges
3 Lean Meat
1 Fat

Calories 212
Calories from Fat. . 115
Total Fat . . . . 13 g
Saturated Fat . . . . . 3.0 g
Cholesterol . . . . 74 mg
Sodium . . . . 62 mg
Total Carbohydrate . . 0 g
Dietary Fiber . . . . 0 g
Sugars . . . . 0 g
Protein . . . . 23 g

Venetian-Style Lamb Chops

4 Servings / Serving Size: 3 lamb chops (1 1/2–2 oz each)

1 Tbsp ground coriander
1 Tbsp ground cinnamon
1 Tbsp ground cumin
1 Tbsp coarsely ground black pepper
Salt to taste
12 loin lamb chops
1 Tbsp olive oil

1 Preheat the oven to 400 degrees. In a small bowl, combine all the spices and the salt. Rub the lamb chops with the spice mixture.

2 Heat the olive oil in a large skillet over medium-high heat. Brown the lamb chops for 2 minutes per side. Transfer the lamb to a roasting pan, place in the oven, and continue to cook for 7–8 minutes or until done as desired.

Exchanges
3 Lean Meat

Calories	176
Calories from Fat	87
Total Fat	10 g
Saturated Fat	2.6 g
Cholesterol	57 mg
Sodium	55 mg
Total Carbohydrate	3 g
Dietary Fiber	2 g
Sugars	0 g
Protein	19 g

Pasta

Angel Hair Pasta with Shrimp and Spinach

4 Servings / Serving Size: 4 oz shrimp, 2 oz cooked pasta

1 lb peeled and deveined large shrimp
1/2 tsp salt
1/4 tsp fresh ground black pepper
1 1/2 Tbsp olive oil
2 small shallots, minced

8 oz angel hair pasta
2 Tbsp lemon juice
1/2 cup low-fat, reduced-sodium chicken broth
2 Tbsp capers
1 cup fresh, cleaned spinach leaves

1 Bring a pot of water to boil.

2 Meanwhile, season the shrimp with salt and pepper. Heat the oil in a large skillet until the oil shimmers. Add the shrimp to the skillet and sauté for about 2 minutes per side. Remove the shrimp from the skillet. Add the shallots to the skillet and sauté for 2 minutes.

3 Add the pasta to the pot of boiling water and cook for 3–4 minutes.

4 Meanwhile, add the lemon juice and broth to the skillet and bring to a boil. Drain the pasta and add it to the skillet. Add the shrimp to the pasta and cook for 30 seconds. Add the capers and spinach leaves and cook just until the spinach wilts, about 1 minute.

Exchanges

3 Starch
2 Very Lean Meat
1/2 Fat

Calories	335
Calories from Fat	61
Total Fat	7 g
Saturated Fat	1.0 g
Cholesterol	131 mg
Sodium	639 mg
Total Carbohydrate	45 g
Dietary Fiber	3 g
Sugars	3 g
Protein	22 g

Asparagus and Shrimp Pasta Toss

4 Servings / Serving Size: 1 cup

8 oz whole wheat shaped
pasta
2 tsp olive oil
2 garlic cloves, minced
1/2 cup chopped red onion
1 1/2 cups diagonally sliced
asparagus, tough ends
removed

3 Tbsp dry white wine
1 15-oz can diced tomatoes
with Italian herbs
2 Tbsp freshly grated Parmesan
cheese

1 Cook the pasta according to the package directions.

2 Meanwhile, heat the oil in a large skillet over medium-high heat.
Add the garlic and onion and sauté for 4 minutes. Add the
asparagus and sauté for 2 minutes.

3 Add the white wine and
simmer on medium heat for
3 minutes. Add the tomatoes and
simmer for 4 minutes.

4 Drain the pasta and add to the
skillet. Toss well. Top each
serving with a sprinkle of Parmesan
cheese.

Exchanges
3 Starch
2 Vegetable
1/2 Fat

Calories 315
  Calories from Fat . . . 44
Total Fat . . . . 5 g
  Saturated Fat . . . . . 1.0 g
Cholesterol . . . . 3 mg
Sodium . . . . 582 mg
Total Carbohydrate . 57 g
  Dietary Fiber . . . . . . 5 g
  Sugars . . . . 11 g
Protein . . . . 12 g

Caramelized Onions and Fusilli

4 Servings / Serving Size: 1 cup

2 Tbsp olive oil
2 large onions, halved and thinly sliced
1/2 cup water
8 oz fusilli pasta

1/2 cup dry white wine
2 Tbsp freshly grated Parmesan cheese
1 Tbsp minced parsley

1 Heat the oil in a large skillet over medium heat. Add the onions and sauté for 10 minutes until they start to brown. Add the water and bring to a boil. Lower the heat, cover, and simmer for 10 minutes until the water is evaporated and the onions are deep brown.

2 Meanwhile, cook the fusilli according to the package directions.

3 Add the white wine to the onions and heat on high until the wine evaporates.

4 Add the cooked pasta to the onions and toss well.

5 Add in the cheese and parsley.

Exchanges
2 1/2 Starch
2 Vegetable
1 1/2 Fat

Calories	330
Calories from Fat	80
Total Fat	9 g
Saturated Fat	1.5 g
Cholesterol	3 mg
Sodium	29 mg
Total Carbohydrate	51 g
Dietary Fiber	4 g
Sugars	9 g
Protein	9 g

Farfalle with Spinach and Cherry Tomatoes

4 Servings / Serving Size: 1 cup

8 oz farfalle (bow tie) noodles
2 tsp olive oil
2 garlic cloves, minced
1/4 tsp crushed red pepper
2 cups halved cherry tomatoes

1/2 cup reduced-sodium, low-fat chicken broth
1 Tbsp chopped basil
2 cups fresh baby spinach
3 Tbsp grated Parmesan cheese

1 Cook the farfalle according to the package directions.

2 Meanwhile, heat the oil in a nonstick skillet over medium-high heat. Add the garlic and red pepper and sauté for 20 seconds.

3 Add the tomatoes, broth, basil, and spinach to the pan and cook for 2 minutes. Drain the pasta and toss with the vegetables. Sprinkle with Parmesan cheese.

Exchanges
3 Starch
1 Vegetable
1/2 Fat

Calories 274
 Calories from Fat . . . 43
Total Fat . . . . 5 g
 Saturated Fat . . . . . 1.2 g
Cholesterol . . . . 4 mg
Sodium . . . . 119 mg
Total Carbohydrate . 47 g
 Dietary Fiber . . . . 3 g
 Sugars . . . . 6 g
Protein . . . . 10 g

Fettuccine with Prosciutto and Asparagus

4 Servings / Serving Size: 1 cup

1 lb fresh asparagus
8 oz fettuccine
1 Tbsp olive oil
1 small onion, minced
2 tsp minced garlic
3 oz chopped lean prosciutto

2 tsp balsamic vinegar
Salt and fresh ground black pepper to taste
1/8 tsp crushed red pepper
2 Tbsp freshly grated Parmesan cheese

1 Break off the woody ends of the asparagus. Diagonally slice each spear into thirds.

2 Add the pasta to a large pot of boiling water and cook for 5–6 minutes. Add the asparagus and cook for 3–4 minutes more until the pasta is tender. Drain and set aside.

3 In the same pot, heat the oil over medium heat. Add the onion and garlic and sauté for 2 minutes. Add the prosciutto and sauté for 2 minutes more. Add the balsamic vinegar and cook 1 more minute. Add the fettuccine and asparagus. Toss with salt, pepper, and crushed red pepper. Top with Parmesan cheese.

Exchanges

2 1/2 Starch
1 Vegetable
1 Lean Meat
1 Fat

Calories 327
  Calories from Fat . . . 78
Total Fat . . . . 9 g
  Saturated Fat . . . . . 2.5 g
Cholesterol . . . . 71 mg
Sodium . . . . 615 mg
Total Carbohydrate . 46 g
  Dietary Fiber . . . . . . 3 g
  Sugars . . . . 5 g
Protein . . . . 17 g

Fusilli and Swordfish

4 Servings / Serving Size: 1 cup

8 oz whole wheat fusilli
noodles
8 oz fresh swordfish steak
Salt and pepper to taste
1 Tbsp olive oil
1 small onion, chopped

2 garlic cloves, minced
1/2 cup dry white wine
1/4 cup minced parsley
1 Tbsp lemon juice
1 tsp fresh oregano, chopped

1 Boil the noodles according to the package directions.

2 Meanwhile, sprinkle the swordfish steak with salt and pepper. Heat
the olive oil in a large nonstick skillet over medium-high heat. Add
the swordfish and sauté for 5 minutes per side. Remove the fish from the
skillet and cut it into cubes.

3 Add the onion and garlic to
the pan. Sauté for 4 minutes.
Add the white wine and bring to a
boil. Reduce for 1 minute. Add the
parsley and lemon juice. Cook for
1 minute. Add the oregano.

4 Drain the pasta, reserving
about 1/4 cup of the pasta
cooking water. Add the water to the
sauce and cook for 2 minutes.

5 Toss the pasta with the sauce
and fold in the swordfish cubes.

Exchanges

3 Starch
1 Vegetable
1 Lean Meat
1/2 Fat

Calories 337
　Calories from Fat. . . 65
Total Fat . . . . .7 g
　Saturated Fat . . . . . 1.2 g
Cholesterol . . . . 22 mg
Sodium . . . . 61 mg
Total Carbohydrate . 46 g
　Dietary Fiber . . . . 4 g
　Sugars . . . . 5 g
Protein. . . . . 19 g

Fusilli with Broccoli, Peppers, and Asiago

4 Servings / Serving Size: 1 cup

8 oz uncooked fusilli or other shaped pasta
1 cup broccoli florets
1 cup sliced red pepper
2 tsp olive oil
1 small shallot, minced
1 1/2 oz grated Asiago cheese
1/4 tsp crushed red pepper flakes
1/4 tsp fresh ground black pepper

1 Cook the pasta for about 10 minutes in a pot of boiling water. During the last 3 minutes, add the broccoli and red pepper.

2 While the pasta and vegetables cook, heat the oil in a small skillet. Add the shallot and sauté for 3 minutes.

3 Drain the pasta and vegetables. Toss the pasta and vegetables in a bowl with the sautéed shallot. Add the Asiago cheese, crushed red pepper, and black pepper and toss well.

Exchanges
2 1/2 Starch
1 Vegetable
1 Fat

Calories 281
  Calories from Fat. . . 61
Total Fat . . . . 7 g
  Saturated Fat . . . . . 2.7 g
Cholesterol . . . . 11 mg
Sodium . . . . 125 mg
Total Carbohydrate . 45 g
  Dietary Fiber . . . . . . 3 g
  Sugars . . . . 4 g
Protein . . . . 11 g

Linguine Alla Caprese

4 Servings / Serving Size: 1 cup

- **8** oz whole wheat linguine
- **2** cups halved cherry tomatoes
- **1/2** red onion, diced
- **2 1/2** oz part-skim mozzarella cheese, cubed into 1/2-inch pieces
- **3** Tbsp minced fresh basil
- **2** Tbsp red wine vinegar
- **1** Tbsp olive oil

1 Cook the noodles according to the package directions.

2 Meanwhile, combine the remaining ingredients in a large bowl. Drain the pasta and add it to the bowl. Toss well and serve.

Exchanges
3 Starch
1 Vegetable
1 Fat

Calories	308
Calories from Fat	72
Total Fat	8 g
Saturated Fat	2.5 g
Cholesterol	10 mg
Sodium	94 mg
Total Carbohydrate	48 g
Dietary Fiber	4 g
Sugars	5 g
Protein	12 g

Linguine with Clams

4 Servings / Serving Size: 1 cup

   8 oz uncooked linguine
1 1/2 Tbsp olive oil
   1 small shallot, minced
   3 garlic cloves, minced
   2 lb small clams in their shells, scrubbed
1/2 cup minced parsley

1 In a large pot of water, cook the linguine for about 9 minutes or until al dente (still slightly firm) and then drain.

2 Meanwhile, heat the oil in a large skillet over medium heat. Add the shallot and garlic and sauté for 2 minutes. Add the clams, cover, and cook for 4 minutes until the clams open their shells; discard any unopened clams. Add in the parsley.

3 Add the linguine to the clams and cook for 1 minute. Transfer to a bowl and serve immediately.

Exchanges
3 Starch
1 Very Lean Meat
1 Fat

Calories 314
  Calories from Fat. . . 61
Total Fat . . . . 7 g
  Saturated Fat . . . . . 0.9 g
Cholesterol . . . . 23 mg
Sodium . . . . 46 mg
Total Carbohydrate . 46 g
  Dietary Fiber . . . . 2 g
  Sugars . . . . 5 g
Protein . . . . 16 g

No Cook Tomato Sauce for Pasta

3 Servings / Serving Size: 1/2 cup

5 large ripe tomatoes, peeled and seeded
2 Tbsp minced fresh basil
1 garlic clove, minced
2 Tbsp olive oil
1 tsp balsamic vinegar
  Salt and pepper to taste

1 Coarsely chop 4 of the tomatoes and place them in a food processor or blender. Add the basil and garlic and puree until smooth. Add the olive oil and puree again.

2 Chop the remaining tomato and fold it in by hand. Drizzle in the balsamic vinegar and season with salt and pepper. Served over cooked pasta or use as a sauce for cooked meats, poultry, or seafood.

Exchanges
2 Vegetable
2 Fat

Calories 137
  Calories from Fat. . . 89
Total Fat . . . . 10 g
  Saturated Fat . . . . . 1.2 g
Cholesterol . . . . 0 mg
Sodium . . . . 23 mg
Total Carbohydrate . 13 g
  Dietary Fiber . . . . 3 g
  Sugars . . . . 8 g
Protein . . . . 2 g

Orecchiette with Broccoli, Bacon, and Garlic

4 Servings / Serving Size: 1 cup

2 slices bacon, chopped	**8** oz uncooked orecchiette pasta or small shells
2 cloves garlic, minced	
2 Tbsp freshly grated Parmesan cheese	**1** 10-oz package frozen broccoli florets, slightly thawed
2/3 cup fat-free ricotta cheese	**1/2** cup drained bottled roasted red peppers, cut into strips
1/4 tsp fresh ground black pepper	**2** Tbsp minced parsley

1 Bring a pot of water to boil for the pasta. Meanwhile, cook the bacon in a medium skillet over medium-high heat. Drain the bacon and remove. Add the garlic and sauté for 30 seconds. Put the garlic and the bacon in a large bowl. Add the cheeses and black pepper and mix well.

2 Cook the orecchiette pasta in the boiling water for about 7 minutes. Add the broccoli and continue to cook for 3 minutes until the pasta is al dente (cooked but still firm). Drain, reserving 1/2 cup of the cooking water. Add the pasta to the bacon and cheese mixture. Add the reserved pasta cooking water and toss well until the pasta and broccoli are coated. Add the red peppers and parsley and toss again.

Exchanges

3 Starch
1 Vegetable
1 Lean Meat

Calories	297
Calories from Fat	34
Total Fat	4 g
Saturated Fat	1.1 g
Cholesterol	18 mg
Sodium	162 mg
Total Carbohydrate	49 g
Dietary Fiber	3 g
Sugars	5 g
Protein	17 g

Pancetta Penne*

4 Servings / Serving Size: 1 cup

    8 oz uncooked penne noodles
1 1/2 oz pancetta bacon, chopped
    1 small onion, chopped
    1 garlic clove, minced
2 1/2 cups marinara sauce
    2 Tbsp chopped black olives
    2 tsp capers
    2 Tbsp grated fresh Parmesan cheese

1 Boil the pasta according to the package directions.

2 Meanwhile, sauté the pancetta, onion, and garlic in a large nonstick skillet for 5 minutes over medium-high heat. Add the marinara sauce and cook for 5 minutes.

3 Add the olives and capers. Add the cooked penne pasta, toss well, and serve with Parmesan cheese.

Exchanges
3 Starch
3 Vegetable
2 Fat

Calories 392
  Calories from Fat . . 108
Total Fat . . . . 12 g
  Saturated Fat . . . . . 3.1 g
Cholesterol . . . . 16 mg
Sodium . . . . 979 mg
Total Carbohydrate . 57 g
  Dietary Fiber . . . . 8 g
  Sugars . . . . 11 g
Protein . . . . 14 g

Note: This recipe has a high sodium content.

Pasta with Cauliflower

4 Servings / Serving Size: 1 cup

8 oz whole wheat pasta (spaghetti or shaped)
1 cup cauliflower
1 tsp olive oil
1 medium onion, chopped
1 slice lean bacon, cut into small pieces
1/4 cup low-fat, reduced-sodium chicken broth
3 Tbsp unseasoned bread crumbs
Dash red pepper flakes
Fresh ground pepper to taste

1 Cook the pasta according to the package directions. During the last minute of cooking, add the cauliflower. Drain and set aside.

2 Heat the olive oil in a large skillet. Add the onion and bacon and sauté for 4 minutes. Add in the bread crumbs, broth, red pepper flakes, and fresh ground pepper.

3 Add in the pasta and cauliflower. Toss well.

Exchanges

3 Starch
1 Vegetable
1 Fat

Calories	293
Calories from Fat	57
Total Fat	6 g
Saturated Fat	1.5 g
Cholesterol	4 mg
Sodium	129 mg
Total Carbohydrate	50 g
Dietary Fiber	4 g
Sugars	5 g
Protein	9 g

Pasta with No Cook Tomato and Pepper Sauce

4 Servings / Serving Size: 1 cup

2 cups cherry tomatoes, halved
3 garlic cloves, finely chopped
1 red pepper, seeded and chopped
1 yellow pepper, seeded and chopped
2 Tbsp minced fresh basil
2 Tbsp olive oil
2 Tbsp red wine vinegar
   Pinch crushed red pepper
   Salt and pepper to taste
8 oz whole wheat pasta

1 Combine the tomatoes, garlic, red and yellow peppers, basil, olive oil, vinegar, crushed red pepper, salt, and pepper. Mix well.

2 Cook the pasta according to the package directions. Drain and toss with the tomato and pepper sauce.

Exchanges
2 1/2 Starch
2 Vegetable
1 1/2 Fat

Calories	310
Calories from Fat	78
Total Fat	9 g
Saturated Fat	1.1 g
Cholesterol	0 mg
Sodium	13 mg
Total Carbohydrate	51 g
Dietary Fiber	5 g
Sugars	8 g
Protein	9 g

Pasta with Roasted Pepper, Onion, and Vermouth

4 Servings / Serving Size: 1 cup

1 8-oz package penne noodles
2 tsp olive oil
1 medium onion, halved and thinly sliced
2 tsp bottled minced garlic
1 7-oz jar roasted red peppers, drained and thinly sliced
1 7-oz jar roasted yellow peppers, drained and thinly sliced

1/2 cup sweet red vermouth
1/4 tsp salt
1/4 tsp fresh black pepper
1/4 tsp dried basil
1/8 tsp crushed red pepper
2 Tbsp freshly grated Parmesan cheese

1 Boil the noodles according to the package directions.

2 Meanwhile, heat the oil in a large skillet over medium-high heat. Add the onion and garlic and sauté for 5 minutes. Add the roasted red and yellow peppers and sauté for 2 minutes. Add the vermouth and cook until the liquid is reduced by half.

3 Add the salt, black pepper, basil, and red pepper. Drain the pasta, reserving 3 Tbsp of cooking liquid. Add the pasta to the pepper mixture and then add the reserved pasta liquid to loosen up the sauce. Cook 1 minute. Top each serving with Parmesan cheese.

Exchanges
3 Starch
1 Vegetable
1/2 Fat

Calories	300
Calories from Fat	41
Total Fat	5 g
Saturated Fat	0.9 g
Cholesterol	3 mg
Sodium	286 mg
Total Carbohydrate	52 g
Dietary Fiber	4 g
Sugars	10 g
Protein	10 g

Pasta with Tuna and Pine Nuts

4 Servings / Serving Size: 1 cup

8 oz whole wheat penne noodles
1/4 cup dried currants
1 Tbsp olive oil
1/2 onion, chopped
2 garlic cloves, minced
2 Tbsp pine nuts
1 small zucchini, halved and thinly sliced

1 carrot, peeled and diced
1/2 cup dry white wine
1 Tbsp tomato paste
1 tsp dried oregano
1 7-oz can water-packed tuna, drained
Salt and pepper to taste

1 Cook the pasta according to the package directions.

2 Place the currants in a small bowl and cover them with boiling water. Let stand for 10 minutes.

3 Meanwhile, heat the olive oil in a large skillet over medium heat. Add the onion and garlic and sauté for 4 minutes. Add the pine nuts and sauté until they turn light brown, about 3 minutes. Remove the onion and nut mixture from the pan.

4 Add the zucchini and carrot and sauté for 3 minutes. Mix the white wine, tomato paste, and oregano and add them to the pan. Cook for 2 minutes. Add the tuna, salt, and pepper and cook for 1 minute.

5 Drain the pasta, reserving 2/3 cup of the cooking liquid. Add the cooking liquid to the tuna. Cook for 1 minute.

6 Toss the pasta with the tuna. Add the onion and pine nut mixture. Drain the currants and add them to the pasta and toss well.

Exchanges	
3 Starch	1 Very Lean Meat
1/2 Fruit	1 Fat
1 Vegetable	

Calories 367	
Calories from Fat . . . 71	
Total Fat . . . . 8 g	
Saturated Fat . . . . . 1.1 g	
Cholesterol . . . . 14 mg	
Sodium . . . . 46 mg	
Total Carbohydrate . 56 g	
Dietary Fiber . . . . 5 g	
Sugars . . . . 13 g	
Protein . . . . 17 g	

Penne with Asparagus
and Baby Spinach

4 Servings / Serving Size: 1 cup

8 oz whole wheat penne pasta
2 tsp olive oil
2 garlic cloves, minced
1 small onion, halved and thinly sliced
1 cup asparagus tips

1/4 tsp crushed red pepper flakes
1/3 cup low-fat, reduced-sodium chicken broth
1 cup baby spinach leaves
2 Tbsp freshly grated Parmesan cheese

1 Cook the pasta according to the package directions.

2 Meanwhile, heat the oil in a large skillet over medium-high heat. Add the garlic and onion and sauté for 4 minutes. Add the asparagus tips and sauté for 4 minutes.

3 Add the crushed red pepper flakes and broth and bring to a boil. Lower the heat and simmer for 3 minutes. Add the spinach and cook until the spinach wilts, about 1 minute.

4 Drain the pasta and toss it with the asparagus mixture. Top each serving with Parmesan cheese.

Exchanges

3 Starch
1/2 Fat

Calories	268
Calories from Fat	44
Total Fat	5 g
Saturated Fat	0.9 g
Cholesterol	3 mg
Sodium	81 mg
Total Carbohydrate	47 g
Dietary Fiber	4 g
Sugars	5 g
Protein	10 g

Penne with Creamy Cheese Sauce

4 Servings / Serving Size: 1 cup

1/4 cup freshly grated Parmesan cheese
1/4 cup fat-free ricotta cheese
  3 Tbsp olive oil
  2 garlic cloves, minced
  8 oz penne noodles
    Salt and pepper to taste

1 In a bowl, combine the cheeses, oil, and garlic.

2 Cook the penne according to the package directions, drain, and reserve 3 Tbsp of the cooking water.

3 Add the cooking water to the cheese mixture and then add the drained noodles and toss well. Season with salt and pepper if desired.

Exchanges
3 Starch
3 Fat

Calories	380
Calories from Fat	158
Total Fat	18 g
Saturated Fat	3.7 g
Cholesterol	10 mg
Sodium	69 mg
Total Carbohydrate	44 g
Dietary Fiber	2 g
Sugars	3 g
Protein	11 g

Quick Italian Sun-Dried Tomato Pasta

4 Servings / Serving Size: 1 cup

8 oz fusilli pasta
1 cup rehydrated, sliced sun-dried tomatoes
1 15-oz can artichoke hearts, halved
1/2 cup pitted Kalamata olives
2 Tbsp minced basil
2 Tbsp Italian parsley

DRESSING

2 Tbsp olive oil
2 Tbsp balsamic vinegar
1 Tbsp lemon juice
 Salt and pepper to taste

1 Cook the noodles according to the package directions, but omit the salt and oil. Drain.

2 Add the tomatoes, artichoke hearts, olives, basil, and parsley to the pasta. Mix together the dressing ingredients, add the dressing to the pasta, and toss well. Serve at room temperature.

Exchanges
3 Starch
2 Vegetable

Calories 281
 Calories from Fat . . . 30
Total Fat . . . . 3 g
 Saturated Fat . . . . . 0.4 g
Cholesterol . . . . 0 mg
Sodium . . . . 329 mg
Total Carbohydrate . 54 g
 Dietary Fiber . . . . 5 g
 Sugars . . . . 7 g
Protein . . . . 11 g

Rigatoni with Pancetta

4 Servings / Serving Size: 1 cup

8 oz rigatoni noodles
1/2 Tbsp olive oil
1 oz pancetta (or 1 oz ham), diced
1 medium onion, diced
3/4 cup frozen peas

1 cup low-fat, reduced-sodium chicken broth
1 cup no-salt-added tomato puree
Salt and pepper to taste
2 Tbsp grated Parmesan cheese

1 Prepare the rigatoni according to the package directions.

2 Meanwhile, heat the olive oil in a large skillet over medium heat. Add the pancetta and sauté for 2 minutes. Add the onion and cook for 3 minutes. Add the peas and cook for 2 minutes.

3 Add the chicken broth and bring to a boil. Add the tomato puree and simmer for 10 minutes until reduced by half.

4 Drain the pasta and add it to the sauce. Toss the pasta with the sauce and add salt and pepper if needed. Top each serving with the cheese.

Exchanges
3 Starch
2 Vegetable
1 Fat

Calories 330
  Calories from Fat . . . 54
Total Fat . . . . 6 g
  Saturated Fat . . . . . 1.6 g
Cholesterol . . . . 8 mg
Sodium . . . . 321 mg
Total Carbohydrate . 55 g
  Dietary Fiber . . . . 5 g
  Sugars . . . . 9 g
Protein . . . . 13 g

Rigatoni with Saffron and Zucchini

4 Servings / Serving Size: 1 cup

8 oz whole wheat rigatoni	**2** Tbsp dry white wine
2 tsp olive oil	Large pinch saffron threads
2 garlic cloves, minced	**1 1/2** cups boiling low-fat, reduced-
1/2 medium onion, diced	sodium chicken broth
1 medium zucchini, halved	Salt and pepper to taste
and sliced	

1 Boil the pasta according to the package directions.

2 Meanwhile, heat the olive oil in a large skillet over medium-high heat. Add the garlic and onion and sauté for 3 minutes. Add the zucchini and sauté for 4 minutes. Add the wine and cook for 2 minutes.

3 Dissolve the saffron threads in the boiling chicken broth. Add the broth mixture to the pan and bring to a boil. Lower the heat and simmer for 10 minutes. Season with salt and pepper.

4 Drain the pasta and add it to the sauce. Toss well and serve.

Exchanges
2 1/2 Starch
1 Vegetable
1/2 Fat

Calories	255
Calories from Fat	35
Total Fat	4 g
Saturated Fat	0.5 g
Cholesterol	0 mg
Sodium	198 mg
Total Carbohydrate	46 g
Dietary Fiber	4 g
Sugars	5 g
Protein	9 g

Spaghetti with Tomatoes and Mozzarella

4 Servings / Serving Size: 1 cup

8 oz whole wheat or white
   spaghetti
4 tomatoes, seeded and chopped
2 tsp capers
2 tsp lemon juice
   Salt and pepper to taste

2 tsp olive oil
1/2 onion, chopped
2 garlic cloves, minced
4 oz shredded part skim
   mozzarella cheese
2 Tbsp minced basil

1 Cook the spaghetti according to the package directions.

2 Combine the tomatoes, capers, lemon juice, salt, and pepper. Let stand for 10 minutes.

3 Meanwhile, heat the olive oil in a skillet over medium heat. Add the onion and garlic and sauté for 5 minutes.

4 Drain any accumulated juices from the tomato mixture and reserve. Add the tomato mixture to the skillet and sauté for 4–5 minutes.

5 Drain the spaghetti and add it to the tomato and onion mixture. Add in the reserved juices. Toss well.

6 Add the mozzarella and basil and toss until the cheese has melted.

Exchanges
2 Vegetable
1 Medium-Fat Meat

Calories 341
   Calories from Fat. . . 79
Total Fat . . . . 9 g
   Saturated Fat . . . . . 3.4 g
Cholesterol . . . . 16 mg
Sodium . . . . 193 mg
Total Carbohydrate . 52 g
   Dietary Fiber . . . . 5 g
   Sugars . . . . 8 g
Protein . . . . 15 g

Straw and Hay

4 Servings / Serving Size: 1 cup

4 oz uncooked fettuccine
4 oz uncooked spinach fettuccine
1/2 Tbsp butter
1 tsp minced garlic
2/3 cup fat-free half-and-half
1/2 package (10-oz) frozen peas, thawed
2 Tbsp grated fresh Parmesan cheese
1/4 tsp fresh ground black pepper
4 oz lean cooked ham, cut into thin slices

1 Cook the fettuccine according to the package directions.

2 Meanwhile, melt the butter in a large nonstick skillet over medium heat. Add the garlic and sauté for 1 minute. Add the half-and-half, peas, cheese, and black pepper. Cook for about 4 minutes.

3 Drain the pasta and add it to the skillet with the ham. Toss the fettuccine so that it absorbs the sauce.

Exchanges
3 Starch
1 Lean Meat
1/2 Fat

Calories 322
  Calories from Fat . . . 53
Total Fat . . . . 6 g
  Saturated Fat . . . . . 2.4 g
Cholesterol . . . . 75 mg
Sodium . . . . 374 mg
Total Carbohydrate . 49 g
  Dietary Fiber . . . . 4 g
  Sugars . . . . 7 g
Protein . . . . 17 g

Whole Wheat Fusilli and Tuna

4 Servings / Serving Size: 1 cup

8 oz whole wheat fusilli noodles (or any other whole wheat pasta)
2 tsp olive oil
1 celery stalk, diced
1 small onion, diced
1/2 tsp dried oregano
1 7-oz can water-packed tuna, drained and flaked
1 cup canned diced tomatoes, drained
Salt and pepper to taste

1 Cook the pasta according to the package directions.

2 Meanwhile, heat the oil in a large skillet over medium-high heat. Add the celery and onion and sauté for 3 minutes. Add the oregano and sauté for 1 minute.

3 Add the tuna and cook for 2 minutes. Add the tomatoes and cook for 3 minutes.

4 Drain the pasta and toss with the tuna mixture. Season with salt and pepper.

Exchanges
3 Starch
1 Vegetable
1/2 Fat

Calories 287
  Calories from Fat . . . 37
Total Fat . . . . 4 g
  Saturated Fat . . . . . 0.4 g
Cholesterol . . . . 14 mg
Sodium . . . . 157 mg
Total Carbohydrate . 47 g
  Dietary Fiber . . . . 4 g
  Sugars . . . . 6 g
Protein . . . . 15 g

Whole Wheat Penne with Prosciutto

4 Servings / Serving Size: 1 cup

- **1** tsp olive oil
- **1/2** onion, diced
- **2** garlic cloves, minced
- **2** oz prosciutto, cut 1/2 inch thick, diced into 1/4-inch pieces
- **1** 15-oz can diced tomatoes, drained
- **2** tsp tomato paste
- **2** tsp balsamic vinegar
- **1** tsp sugar
- **8** oz whole wheat penne noodles
- **1** Tbsp freshly grated Parmesan cheese

1 Heat the olive oil in a large skillet over medium-high heat. Add the onion, garlic, and prosciutto and sauté for 4 minutes. Add the tomatoes, tomato paste, vinegar, and sugar and bring to a boil. Lower the heat and simmer for 10 minutes.

2 Meanwhile, boil the noodles according to the package directions. Drain. Toss the pasta with the sauce and top with Parmesan cheese.

Exchanges
3 Starch
1 Vegetable
1/2 Fat

Calories	295
Calories from Fat	56
Total Fat	6 g
Saturated Fat	2.5 g
Cholesterol	16 mg
Sodium	485 mg
Total Carbohydrate	49 g
Dietary Fiber	4 g
Sugars	7 g
Protein	12 g

Other Main Dishes

Fast Pizza with Mozzarella and Sun-Dried Tomatoes

6 Servings / Serving Size: 1/6 of pizza

1 12-inch thin Boboli pizza crust (available in most supermarkets)
2 tsp olive oil
1 tsp dried oregano
1 tsp dried basil
2 cups whole sun-dried tomatoes, rehydrated
3/4 cup reduced-fat mozzarella cheese, shredded
2 Tbsp freshly grated Parmesan cheese

1 Preheat the oven to 400 degrees.

2 Brush the pizza crust with olive oil. Sprinkle with dried oregano and basil. Bake the crust for 10 minutes until crispy.

3 Sprinkle the sun-dried tomatoes and cheeses evenly over the crust. Return the pizza to the oven and bake it until the cheese melts, about 5 minutes. Cut into wedges to serve.

Exchanges
1 1/2 Starch
2 Vegetable
1 Lean Meat
1 Fat

Calories 256
  Calories from Fat. . . 88
Total Fat . . . . 10 g
  Saturated Fat . . . . . 2.5 g
Cholesterol . . . . 23 mg
Sodium . . . . 278 mg
Total Carbohydrate . 33 g
  Dietary Fiber . . . . 3 g
  Sugars . . . . 7 g
Protein . . . . 11 g

Frittata with Onion

4 Servings / Serving Size: 1/4 of frittata

2 eggs
4 egg whites
1 small onion, very finely diced
1 Tbsp minced parsley
1/3 cup frozen peas
3 Tbsp part-skim mozzarella cheese, shredded
Salt and pepper to taste
Nonstick cooking spray

1 Preheat the oven to 350 degrees.

2 In a large bowl, beat together the eggs and egg whites. Add the onion, parsley, peas, and mozzarella cheese. Season with salt and pepper.

3 Spray an ovenproof 10-inch skillet with cooking spray. When the skillet is sizzling, add the egg mixture and cook for 3–4 minutes until the bottom has set.

4 Place the frittata in the oven and bake for 7–9 minutes until cooked through. Cut into wedges to serve.

Exchanges

1 Vegetable
1 Lean Meat

Calories 87
  Calories from Fat . . . 30
Total Fat . . . . 3 g
  Saturated Fat . . . . . 1.3 g
Cholesterol . . . . 109 mg
Sodium . . . . 126 mg
Total Carbohydrate . . 5 g
  Dietary Fiber . . . . 1 g
  Sugars . . . . 3 g
Protein . . . . 9 g

Hot Mushroom Open-Faced Sandwich

4 Servings / Serving Size: 1 sandwich

2 tsp olive oil

2 garlic cloves, minced

2 large portobello mushrooms, cleaned, stemmed, and sliced into 1/2-inch slices

8 oz button mushrooms, cleaned and stemmed

8 oz cremini mushrooms, cleaned and stemmed

1/4 cup low-fat, reduced-sodium beef broth

3 Tbsp dry red wine

2 tsp tomato paste

4 2-oz slices Italian bread

2 Tbsp minced parsley

2 Tbsp grated Parmesan cheese

1 Preheat the oven to 400 degrees. Heat the oil in a large skillet over medium-high heat. Add the garlic and sauté for 1 minute. Add the mushrooms and sauté for 4–5 minutes until they begin to brown.

2 Mix together the beef broth, red wine, and tomato paste. Add the mixture to the mushrooms and cook for 2–3 minutes until it thickens slightly.

3 Place the bread slices on a baking sheet and toast in the oven for 3 minutes. Divide the mushroom mixture among the bread slices and sprinkle with parsley and Parmesan cheese.

4 Return the bread slices to the oven and bake for 2–3 minutes until the cheese is lightly browned. Eat the sandwich with a fork and knife!

Exchanges

2 Starch
1 Vegetable
1 Fat

Calories 238
  Calories from Fat . . . 53
Total Fat . . . . 6 g
  Saturated Fat . . . . . 1.3 g
Cholesterol . . . . 3 mg
Sodium . . . . 391 mg
Total Carbohydrate . 37 g
  Dietary Fiber . . . . 4 g
  Sugars . . . . 5 g
Protein . . . . 10 g

Main Dish Tuscan Bean Salad

4 Servings / Serving Size: 1 1/4 cup

1 small red onion, minced
2 celery stalks, minced
2 medium carrots, diced
3 garlic cloves, minced
1 Tbsp minced fresh basil
1 Tbsp minced fresh mint
2 tsp minced fresh parsley
3 Tbsp fresh lemon juice
1 1/2 Tbsp olive oil
2 15-oz cans cannellini beans or other white beans, drained

Combine the ingredients in order, cover, and refrigerate for a half hour before serving. Serve the salad at room temperature.

Exchanges
2 1/2 Starch
1 Vegetable
1 Fat

Calories	258
Calories from Fat	53
Total Fat	6 g
Saturated Fat	0.8 g
Cholesterol	0 mg
Sodium	188 mg
Total Carbohydrate	40 g
Dietary Fiber	11 g
Sugars	3 g
Protein	13 g

Zucchini Frittata

4 Servings / Serving Size: 1/4 of frittata

2 tsp olive oil
1 large zucchini, thinly sliced
1 garlic clove, minced
Salt and pepper to taste
2 eggs
4 egg whites

1 1/2 Tbsp freshly grated Parmesan cheese
10 basil leaves, torn
1 oz reduced-fat goat cheese, crumbled, or part-skim shredded mozzarella cheese, shredded

1 Preheat the oven to 425. Heat the olive oil in a large ovenproof skillet over medium-high heat. Add the zucchini, garlic, salt, and pepper and sauté for 5 minutes. Remove from the skillet, discarding all but 1 tsp of the oil.

2 Beat together the eggs, egg whites, Parmesan cheese, and basil.

3 Add the egg mixture to the skillet and turn the heat to medium low. Allow the frittata to set without turning it. Add the zucchini mixture and the goat or mozzarella cheese.

4 Cook over medium-low heat for 3 minutes. Transfer the skillet to the oven and cook at 425 degrees for 5–8 minutes. Turn the oven setting to broil and broil for 1–2 minutes until the top is lightly browned. Cut into wedges to serve.

Exchanges
1 Vegetable
1 Lean Meat
1/2 Fat

Calories 112
Calories from Fat. . . 59
Total Fat . . . . 7 g
Saturated Fat . . . . . 2.2 g
Cholesterol . . . . 113 mg
Sodium . . . . 148 mg
Total Carbohydrate . . 4 g
Dietary Fiber . . . . 1 g
Sugars . . . . 2 g
Protein . . . . 10 g

Vegetables (Vendure)

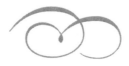

Arugula Salad

4 Servings / Serving Size: 1 cup

1 lb baby arugula leaves
2 oranges, peeled, halved, and sliced
1 small red onion, peeled, halved, and sliced
2 Tbsp toasted slivered almonds

DRESSING

1 garlic clove, minced
2 Tbsp red wine vinegar
1 tsp Dijon mustard
1 Tbsp lemon juice
1 1/2 Tbsp olive oil
Salt and pepper to taste

1 Combine the arugula, oranges, and red onion in a salad bowl.

2 Combine the garlic, red wine vinegar, mustard, and lemon juice in a small bowl. Slowly add the oil and mix well. Add the salt and pepper.

3 Pour the dressing over the salad and top with toasted almonds.

Exchanges
1/2 Fruit
2 Vegetable
1 1/2 Fat

Calories 145
  Calories from Fat . . . 73
Total Fat . . . . 8 g
  Saturated Fat . . . . . 1.0 g
Cholesterol . . . . 0 mg
Sodium . . . . 62 mg
Total Carbohydrate . 17 g
  Dietary Fiber . . . . 4 g
  Sugars . . . . 11 g
Protein . . . . 5 g

Asparagus Salad

4 Servings / Serving Size: about 7 spears, 1 cup greens, about 1 3/4 Tbsp dressing

1 lb asparagus, stems trimmed
1 Tbsp lemon juice
1 tsp olive oil

SALAD

4 cups mixed greens
1 cup halved cherry tomatoes
1 red onion, halved and thinly sliced

DRESSING

3 Tbsp sherry vinegar
1 1/2 Tbsp olive oil
1 Tbsp water
1 tsp Dijon mustard
Salt and pepper to taste

1 Bring a pot of water to boil. Add the asparagus and turn off the heat. Let the asparagus stand in the water for 1 minute. Drain and rinse with cool water. Pat dry. In the bottom of a bowl, combine the lemon juice and olive oil. Add the asparagus and toss to coat.

2 Heat a grill pan on medium-high heat or set an oven broiler to high. Place the asparagus on the grill pan or on a broiler pan lined with foil. Grill or broil the asparagus for about 2 minutes per side until it has grill marks. Remove the asparagus from the grill or broiler.

3 On a platter, add the greens and cherry tomatoes and sprinkle the sliced red onion over them. Top with the asparagus spears.

4 Combine the dressing ingredients and pour over the salad.

Exchanges

2 Vegetable
1 Fat

Calories 98
  Calories from Fat . . . 60
Total Fat . . . . 7 g
  Saturated Fat . . . . . 0.8 g
Cholesterol . . . . 0 mg
Sodium . . . . 48 mg
Total Carbohydrate . . 9 g
  Dietary Fiber . . . . . . 2 g
  Sugars . . . . 5 g
Protein . . . . 2 g

Asparagus with Pine Nuts and Sun-Dried Tomatoes

4 Servings / Serving Size: 2/3 cup

- **1** lb asparagus, bottoms trimmed
- **1** tsp olive oil
- **2** garlic cloves, minced
- **1/2** small onion, minced
- **1/3** cup low-fat, reduced-sodium chicken broth
- **10** sun-dried tomatoes, rehydrated in water, drained, and sliced
- **1** Tbsp pine nuts
  Salt and pepper to taste

1 Slice the asparagus into 2-inch lengths. Heat the oil in a large nonstick skillet. Add the asparagus, garlic, and onion and sauté for 4 minutes. Add the broth and then cover and steam for 3 minutes.

2 Uncover, add the tomatoes and pine nuts, and continue to sauté for 2 minutes more. Season with salt and pepper.

Exchanges
2 Vegetable
1/2 Fat

Calories	61
Calories from Fat	25
Total Fat	3 g
Saturated Fat	0.4 g
Cholesterol	0 mg
Sodium	50 mg
Total Carbohydrate	8 g
Dietary Fiber	2 g
Sugars	4 g
Protein	3 g

Broccoli with Lemon

4 Servings / Serving Size: 2/3 cup

1 tsp olive oil
1 garlic clove, minced
1/2 cup minced red onion
1 lb broccoli, cut into florets, stems peeled and sliced
1/2 cup low-fat, low-sodium chicken broth
2 tsp lemon juice
1 tsp lemon zest

1 Heat the oil in a large nonstick skillet over medium-high heat. Add the garlic and onion and sauté for 3 minutes. Add the broccoli and broth. Cover and steam for 6 minutes.

2 Add the lemon juice and lemon zest and cook, uncovered, for 30 seconds.

Exchanges	
1 Vegetable	

Calories	42
Calories from Fat	12
Total Fat	1 g
Saturated Fat	0.2 g
Cholesterol	0 mg
Sodium	83 mg
Total Carbohydrate	6 g
Dietary Fiber	2 g
Sugars	3 g
Protein	3 g

Broccoli with Red Onion and Pine Nuts

4 Servings / Serving Size: 2/3 cup

1 tsp olive oil
1 medium red onion, halved, peeled, and sliced
1 garlic clove, minced
1 lb broccoli, stems removed and cut into florets
1/2 cup low-fat, reduced-sodium chicken broth
2 Tbsp pine nuts

1 Heat the oil in a large skillet over medium-high heat. Add the red onion and garlic and sauté for 4 minutes. Add the broccoli and sauté for 2 minutes.

2 Add the broth and bring to a boil. Cover, reduce the heat to low, and cook for 4 minutes.

3 Meanwhile, place the pine nuts in a small skillet over medium-high heat and toast them for 3–4 minutes until lightly browned. Sprinkle the pine nuts over the broccoli.

Exchanges
1 Vegetable
1 Fat

Calories	70
Calories from Fat	36
Total Fat	4 g
Saturated Fat	0.7 g
Cholesterol	0 mg
Sodium	83 mg
Total Carbohydrate	8 g
Dietary Fiber	3 g
Sugars	3 g
Protein	4 g

Broccoli with Seasoned Walnuts

4 Servings / Serving Size: 2/3 cup

1/2 tsp olive oil
3 Tbsp walnuts
1/4 tsp paprika
1/4 tsp dried thyme
1/4 tsp dried basil
1/4 tsp dried oregano
Salt and pepper to taste
1 lb broccoli, cut into florets, stems trimmed and sliced
1/3 cup low-fat, reduced-sodium chicken broth

1 Heat the oil in a large nonstick skillet. Add the walnuts and toast over medium heat for 2 minutes. Add the seasonings and continue to sauté for 1–2 minutes. Remove the walnuts from the skillet.

2 Add the broccoli and broth to the skillet. Cover and steam for 4–5 minutes until the broccoli is bright green and crisp. Top the broccoli with the walnuts.

Exchanges
1 Vegetable
1 Fat

Calories	63
Calories from Fat	40
Total Fat	4 g
Saturated Fat	0.4 g
Cholesterol	0 mg
Sodium	60 mg
Total Carbohydrate	5 g
Dietary Fiber	3 g
Sugars	2 g
Protein	3 g

Cauliflower with Crumb Topping

4 Servings / Serving Size: 2/3 cup

1 medium head cauliflower, separated into florets

3 slices (2 oz total) fresh Italian bread

1 garlic clove, crushed and peeled

1 Tbsp Parmesan cheese

1/2 tsp dried oregano

1/2 tsp dried basil

1/4 tsp paprika

1/8 tsp crushed red pepper flakes

Salt and pepper to taste

1 Tbsp olive oil

1 Place the cauliflower in a steamer over boiling water. Cover and steam the cauliflower for 15–18 minutes.

2 Meanwhile, toast the slices of bread in a 400-degree oven or toaster oven for 2 minutes until just the edges begin to brown. Rub the garlic clove over both sides of each piece of bread. Add the bread, cheese, oregano, basil, paprika, red pepper flakes, salt, and pepper to a blender or food processor and process until you have coarse crumbs.

3 Put the crumbs in a bowl and add the olive oil. Mix well.

4 Drain the cauliflower and put it in a serving bowl. Top the cauliflower with the crumbs.

Exchanges
1/2 Starch
2 Vegetable
1/2 Fat

Calories 113
  Calories from Fat. . . 42
Total Fat . . . . 5 g
  Saturated Fat . . . . . 0.8 g
Cholesterol . . . . 1 mg
Sodium . . . . 137 mg
Total Carbohydrate . 15 g
  Dietary Fiber . . . . 4 g
  Sugars . . . . 4 g
Protein . . . . 5 g

Cauliflower with Tomatoes and Peppers

4 Servings / Serving Size: 2/3 cup

1 small head cauliflower, separated into florets
1 tsp olive oil
2 garlic cloves, minced
1/2 small onion, minced
1 cup canned diced no-salt-added tomatoes
1 7-oz jar roasted red peppers in water, drained and diced
1/2 tsp dried oregano
1/2 tsp dried thyme
Salt and pepper to taste

1 Cover and steam the cauliflower for 8–9 minutes in a steamer set above boiling water.

2 Meanwhile, heat the oil in a large skillet over medium-high heat. Add the garlic and onion and sauté for 3 minutes. Add the tomatoes and roasted peppers and sauté for 3 minutes. Add the oregano, thyme, salt, and pepper. Cook for 2 minutes.

3 Drain the cauliflower and add it to the tomato mixture. Cook for 1 minute.

Exchanges
2 Vegetable

Calories 54
  Calories from Fat. . . 14
Total Fat . . . . 2 g
  Saturated Fat . . . . . 0.2 g
Cholesterol . . . . 0 mg
Sodium . . . . 101 mg
Total Carbohydrate . 10 g
  Dietary Fiber . . . . 3 g
  Sugars . . . . 6 g
Protein . . . . 3 g

Fennel and Orange Salad

**4 Servings / Serving Size: 2/3 cup vegetables,
1 cup salad greens, 1 1/4 Tbsp dressing**

2 medium fennel bulbs
1 red onion, peeled, halved, and sliced thin
2 oranges, peeled, halved, and sliced thin
4 cups salad greens

DRESSING

2 1/2 Tbsp white wine vinegar
1 1/2 Tbsp olive oil
1 Tbsp orange juice
1 tsp honey
Salt and pepper to taste

1 Remove the fennel stems and fronds and discard. Cut the bulb end of the fennel into thin strips.

2 Combine the fennel strips, red onion, and oranges in a salad bowl.

3 Combine the dressing ingredients. Add the dressing to the fennel and toss well. Serve at room temperature over salad greens.

Exchanges

1 Fruit
2 Vegetable
1 Fat

Calories 145
  Calories from Fat. . . 50
Total Fat . . . . 6 g
  Saturated Fat . . . . . 0.7 g
Cholesterol . . . . 0 mg
Sodium . . . . 69 mg
Total Carbohydrate . 24 g
  Dietary Fiber . . . . 6 g
  Sugars . . . . 14 g
Protein . . . . 3 g

Garlicky Mushroom Medley

4 Servings / Serving Size: 1/2 cup

2 tsp olive oil
3 garlic cloves, minced
8 oz button mushrooms, cleaned and stemmed
4 oz cremini mushrooms, cleaned and stemmed
4 oz oyster mushrooms, cleaned and stems trimmed
1/3 cup low-fat, reduced-sodium chicken broth
1 tsp fresh lemon juice
1/8 tsp crushed red pepper flakes
    Salt and pepper to taste
1 Tbsp minced parsley

1 Heat the oil in a large nonstick skillet over high heat. Add the garlic and sauté for 30 seconds. Add the mushrooms and sauté for 4–5 minutes until they begin to release their juices and turn brown.

2 Add the broth, lemon juice, crushed red pepper, salt, and pepper. Bring to a boil. Lower the heat and cook until the broth has evaporated.

3 Sprinkle with parsley.

Exchanges
1 Vegetable
1/2 Fat

Calories	53
Calories from Fat	25
Total Fat	3 g
Saturated Fat	0.3 g
Cholesterol	0 mg
Sodium	48 mg
Total Carbohydrate	6 g
Dietary Fiber	1 g
Sugars	2 g
Protein	3 g

Grated Zucchini and Yellow Squash Salad

4 Servings / Serving Size: 1/2 cup

SALAD

1/2 medium zucchini, unpeeled and shredded

1/2 medium yellow squash, unpeeled and shredded

1 large carrot, peeled and shredded

1/2 large red pepper, diced

3 Tbsp minced parsley

DRESSING

3 Tbsp red wine vinegar

1 Tbsp lemon juice

1 tsp Dijon mustard

2 Tbsp olive oil

1 garlic clove, finely minced
Salt and pepper to taste

1 Combine the salad ingredients in a large salad bowl.

2 Whisk together the vinegar, lemon juice, and mustard. Slowly pour in the oil, whisking constantly. Stir in the garlic, salt, and pepper and whisk again. Pour the dressing over the salad and serve.

Exchanges
1 Vegetable
1 1/2 Fat

Calories	91
Calories from Fat	63
Total Fat	7 g
Saturated Fat	0.9 g
Cholesterol	0 mg
Sodium	53 mg
Total Carbohydrate	7 g
Dietary Fiber	2 g
Sugars	4 g
Protein	1 g

Green Beans with Lemon

4 Servings / Serving Size: 1/2 cup

1 lb fresh green beans, trimmed
1 tsp olive oil
1 garlic clove, minced
2 tsp lemon zest
1 Tbsp fresh lemon juice
1/4 cup low-fat, reduced-sodium chicken broth
1 tsp dried thyme
Salt and pepper to taste

1 Steam the green beans for 5–6 minutes in a steamer set above boiling water.

2 Meanwhile, heat the oil in a large nonstick skillet. Add the garlic and sauté for 1 minute. Add the remaining ingredients and bring to a boil. Drain the green beans and add them to the lemon and chicken broth mixture. Cook for 2 minutes.

Exchanges
2 Vegetable

Calories 47
 Calories from Fat . . . 13
Total Fat . . . . 1 g
 Saturated Fat . . . . . 0.2 g
Cholesterol . . . . 0 mg
Sodium . . . . 35 mg
Total Carbohydrate . . 8 g
 Dietary Fiber . . . . 3 g
 Sugars . . . . 2 g
Protein . . . . 2 g

Green Beans with Sautéed Onions

4 Servings / Serving Size: 1/2 cup

2 tsp olive oil
1 medium red onion, halved and sliced thin
2 garlic cloves, minced
1/2 tsp dried thyme
1/2 tsp dried oregano
1 lb green beans, trimmed
1/3 cup low-fat, reduced-sodium chicken broth
1 Tbsp toasted pine nuts

1 Heat the oil in a large skillet over medium heat. Add the onion and garlic and sauté for 5 minutes. Add the thyme and oregano and sauté for 2 minutes.

2 Add the green beans and broth. Cover and steam for 4 minutes until the green beans are bright green and crisp. Top with toasted pine nuts.

Exchanges
2 Vegetable
1/2 Fat

Calories	82
Calories from Fat	35
Total Fat	4 g
Saturated Fat	0.6 g
Cholesterol	0 mg
Sodium	46 mg
Total Carbohydrate	11 g
Dietary Fiber	4 g
Sugars	3 g
Protein	3 g

Green Beans with Tomatoes and Herbs

4 Servings / Serving Size: 2/3 cup

1 tsp olive oil
2 garlic cloves, minced
1/2 small onion, diced
1 lb green beans, trimmed
1/2 cup low-fat, reduced-sodium chicken broth
2 plum tomatoes, seeded and diced
2 tsp minced fresh oregano (1 tsp dried)
1 tsp minced fresh thyme (1/2 tsp dried)
　　Salt and pepper to taste

1 Heat the oil in a skillet over medium heat. Add the garlic and onion and sauté for 3 minutes.

2 Add the green beans and sauté for 1 minute. Add the broth, cover, and steam for 5 minutes.

3 Add the tomatoes and herbs, cover, and cook for 2 minutes. Season with salt and pepper.

Exchanges
2 Vegetable

Calories 60
　Calories from Fat . . . 14
Total Fat . . . . 2 g
　Saturated Fat . . . . . 0.2 g
Cholesterol . . . . 0 mg
Sodium . . . . 69 mg
Total Carbohydrate . 11 g
　Dietary Fiber . . . . 4 g
　Sugars . . . . 4 g
Protein . . . . 3 g

Grilled Portobello Mushrooms

4 Servings / Serving Size: 1 mushroom

2 Tbsp balsamic vinegar
1 Tbsp olive oil
2 garlic cloves, finely minced
  Salt and pepper to taste
4 medium portobello mushrooms, cleaned and stemmed

1 In a small bowl, combine the vinegar, oil, garlic, salt, and pepper.

2 Heat a grill pan on high or prepare an outdoor grill on medium-high heat with the rack set 6 inches from the heat source.

3 Add the portobello mushrooms, gill side down, to the hot grill pan or grill rack. Brush the top of the mushrooms with the vinegar and oil mixture. Grill the mushroom for 4–5 minutes and turn. Brush more of the vinegar and oil mixture on the mushroom and continue to grill for 4–5 more minutes until it is cooked through.

Exchanges
1 Vegetable
1/2 Fat

Calories	52
Calories from Fat	33
Total Fat	4 g
Saturated Fat	0.4 g
Cholesterol	0 mg
Sodium	3 mg
Total Carbohydrate	5 g
Dietary Fiber	1 g
Sugars	2 g
Protein	1 g

Grilled Zucchini and Yellow Squash Spears

4 Servings / Serving Size: 2 (approximately 4-inch) pieces

1 large zucchini, unpeeled, halved crosswise and lengthwise
1 large yellow squash, unpeeled, halved crosswise and lengthwise
1 Tbsp olive oil
2 garlic cloves, finely minced
1 tsp dried oregano
1/2 tsp dried thyme
   Salt and pepper

1 Prepare an outdoor grill set to medium high or an oven broiler set to high. Place the zucchini and yellow squash, skin side up, directly on the hot rack or on a broiler tray lined with foil.

2 In a small bowl, combine the remaining ingredients. Brush some of the oil mixture over the zucchini and yellow squash spears and grill for 4–5 minutes. Turn the spears over and brush them again with some of the oil mixture. Grill for another 4–5 minutes until the zucchini and yellow squash are tender.

Exchanges
1 Vegetable
1 Fat

Calories 59
  Calories from Fat. . . 33
Total Fat . . . . 4 g
  Saturated Fat . . . . . 0.5 g
Cholesterol . . . . 0 mg
Sodium . . . . 10 mg
Total Carbohydrate . . 6 g
  Dietary Fiber . . . . 2 g
  Sugars . . . . 4 g
Protein . . . . 2 g

Pepper and Basil Salad

4 Servings / Serving Size: 1/2 cup vegetables, 1 1/4 Tbsp dressing

1 medium red pepper,
seeded, cored, and sliced
into strips
1 medium yellow pepper,
seeded, cored, and sliced
into strips
1/2 medium red onion, diced
2 celery stalks, sliced thin
3 scallions, minced
2 Tbsp minced parsley
16 whole basil leaves

DRESSING
3 Tbsp red wine vinegar
1 1/2 Tbsp olive oil
2 tsp lemon juice
1 tsp Dijon mustard
Salt and pepper to taste

1 For the salad, combine the peppers, onion, celery, scallions, parsley, and basil. Toss well.

2 Combine the dressing ingredients. Pour the dressing over the salad and toss again.

Exchanges
2 Vegetable
1 Fat

Calories 82
  Calories from Fat . . . 48
Total Fat . . . . 5 g
  Saturated Fat . . . . . 0.7 g
Cholesterol . . . . 0 mg
Sodium . . . . 53 mg
Total Carbohydrate . . 9 g
  Dietary Fiber . . . . 2 g
  Sugars . . . . 4 g
Protein . . . . 1 g

Peppers and Onions

4 Servings / Serving Size: 1/2 cup

1 tsp olive oil
1 medium onion, halved and sliced into strips
2 garlic cloves, minced
1 medium red pepper, seeded, cored, and sliced into thin strips
1 medium yellow pepper, seeded, cored, and sliced into thin strips

1 medium green pepper, seeded, cored, and sliced into thin strips
2 tsp fresh minced fresh oregano
1/3 cup low-fat, reduced-sodium chicken broth
Salt and pepper to taste

1 Heat the oil in a large skillet over medium-high heat. Add the onion and garlic and sauté for 5 minutes.

2 Add the peppers and sauté for 5 minutes until they begin to soften. Add the oregano, broth, salt, and pepper. Cover and steam for 3 minutes.

Exchanges
2 Vegetable

Calories	55
Calories from Fat	13
Total Fat	1 g
Saturated Fat	0.2 g
Cholesterol	0 mg
Sodium	46 mg
Total Carbohydrate	10 g
Dietary Fiber	3 g
Sugars	6 g
Protein	2 g

Roasted Asparagus

4 Servings / Serving Size: 5 spears

20 medium-width asparagus spears
 2 tsp olive oil
 2 tsp lemon juice
   Salt and pepper to taste
 2 garlic cloves, very finely minced

1 Preheat the oven to 450 degrees.

2 Place the asparagus spears side by side in a single layer on a baking sheet lined with parchment paper or aluminum foil sprayed with cooking spray.

3 Combine the remaining ingredients and sprinkle them over the asparagus.

4 Roast the asparagus for 10 minutes until cooked through but crisp.

Exchanges
1 Vegetable
1/2 Fat

Calories	41
Calories from Fat	23
Total Fat	3 g
Saturated Fat	0.3 g
Cholesterol	0 mg
Sodium	9 mg
Total Carbohydrate	4 g
Dietary Fiber	1 g
Sugars	2 g
Protein	2 g

Roasted Herb Potatoes

4 Servings / Serving Size: 1/2 medium potato

2 medium Yukon gold potatoes, unpeeled and cut into 1-inch cubes
2 tsp olive oil
4 rosemary sprigs
2 garlic cloves, minced
   Salt and pepper to taste

1 Preheat the oven to 450 degrees. Bring a pot of water to boil. Add the potatoes and boil for 5 minutes. Drain.

2 Tear aluminum foil into four 3 × 3-inch squares. Divide the potatoes evenly among all the squares. Drizzle each potato packet with olive oil. Top with a rosemary sprig and some garlic. Sprinkle with salt and pepper. Fold each packet tightly.

3 Roast the packet for 25 minutes until potatoes are cooked through.

Exchanges
1 Starch

Calories 84	
Calories from Fat . . . 21	
Total Fat . . . . 2 g	
Saturated Fat . . . . . 0.3 g	
Cholesterol . . . . 0 mg	
Sodium . . . . 3 mg	
Total Carbohydrate . 15 g	
Dietary Fiber . . . . 1 g	
Sugars . . . . 2 g	
Protein . . . . 1 g	

Sautéed Arugula with Slivered Garlic

4 Servings / Serving Size: 2/3 cup

2 tsp olive oil
3 garlic cloves, peeled and thinly sliced
2 lb baby arugula leaves
Salt and pepper to taste

Heat the oil in a large nonstick skillet. Add the garlic and sauté for 30 seconds. Add the arugula leaves and sauté until the leaves just wilt, about 3–4 minutes. Sprinkle with salt and pepper.

Exchanges
2 Vegetable
1/2 Fat

Calories 80
 Calories from Fat . . . 34
Total Fat . . . . 4 g
 Saturated Fat . . . . . 0.5 g
Cholesterol . . . . 0 mg
Sodium . . . . 62 mg
Total Carbohydrate . . 9 g
 Dietary Fiber . . . . 4 g
 Sugars . . . . 5 g
Protein . . . . 6 g

Sautéed Fennel

4 Servings / Serving Size: 2/3 cup

  2 medium fennel bulbs
  2 tsp olive oil
  2 medium carrots, peeled and julienned
  1 medium onion, halved, peeled, and sliced thin
1/2 cup low-fat, reduced-sodium chicken broth
  1 tsp dried thyme
     Salt and pepper to taste

1 Remove the stems and fronds from the fennel bulb. Cut the bulb into thick strips.

2 Heat the oil in a large nonstick skillet over medium-high heat. Add the carrots and onion and sauté for 6 minutes. Add the fennel and sauté for 4 minutes. Add the broth, thyme, salt, and pepper and bring to a boil. Lower the heat, cover, and simmer for 5 minutes. Uncover and raise the heat to evaporate the liquid, about 2 minutes.

Exchanges
3 Vegetable
1/2 Fat

Calories 94	
Calories from Fat . . . 24	
Total Fat . . . . 3 g	
Saturated Fat . . . . . 0.3 g	
Cholesterol . . . . 0 mg	
Sodium . . . . 159 mg	
Total Carbohydrate . 17 g	
Dietary Fiber . . . . 6 g	
Sugars . . . . 7 g	
Protein . . . . 3 g	

Spinach Salad with Balsamic Dressing

4 Servings / Serving Size: 1 cup salad, 1 1/4 Tbsp dressing

4 cups baby spinach leaves, cleaned
1 medium red onion, halved and sliced thin
1 Granny Smith apple, halved and sliced thin
3 Tbsp Gorgonzola cheese

DRESSING
3 Tbsp balsamic vinegar
1 1/2 Tbsp olive oil
2 tsp lemon juice
1/2 tsp Dijon mustard

1 In a salad bowl, combine the spinach, red onion, and apple.

2 Whisk together the dressing ingredients, pour them over the salad, and toss well.

3 Garnish the salad with the cheese.

Exchanges

1/2 Fruit
1 Vegetable
1 Fat

Calories 107
 Calories from Fat . . . 58
Total Fat . . . . 6 g
 Saturated Fat . . . . . 1.4 g
Cholesterol . . . . 3 mg
Sodium . . . . 100 mg
Total Carbohydrate . 12 g
 Dietary Fiber . . . . 2 g
 Sugars . . . . 7 g
Protein . . . . 2 g

Spinach with Garlic and Leeks

4 Servings / Serving Size: 1/2 cup

- **2** tsp olive oil
- **4** garlic cloves, minced
- **1** leek, white bottom part only, cleaned and sliced thin
- **1/8** tsp crushed red pepper flakes
- **3** lb fresh baby spinach leaves, cleaned
  Salt and pepper to taste

1 Heat the oil in a large skillet over medium-high heat. Add the garlic and the leek and sauté for 5 minutes. Add the crushed red pepper and sauté for 1 minute.

2 Add the spinach and cook for 2–4 minutes until it just wilts and before it starts to give off too much liquid. Season with salt and pepper.

Exchanges
3 Vegetable
1 Fat

Calories	117
Calories from Fat	31
Total Fat	3 g
Saturated Fat	0.3 g
Cholesterol	0 mg
Sodium	278 mg
Total Carbohydrate	16 g
Dietary Fiber	10 g
Sugars	3 g
Protein	11 g

Tomato and Basil Salad

4 Servings / Serving Size: about 2/3 cup salad, 1 1/4 Tbsp dressing

- **2** cups halved cherry tomatoes
- **2** plum tomatoes, seeded and diced
- **2** Tbsp minced chives
- **10** basil leaves

DRESSING
- **2** Tbsp red wine vinegar
- **1 1/2** Tbsp olive oil
- **2** tsp lemon juice
- **1** tsp Dijon mustard

1 Combine the tomatoes and chives and place on a platter.

2 Whisk together the dressing ingredients and drizzle them over the salad.

3 Top the salad with the basil leaves.

Exchanges
1 Vegetable
1 Fat

Calories	71
Calories from Fat	49
Total Fat	5 g
Saturated Fat	0.7 g
Cholesterol	0 mg
Sodium	40 mg
Total Carbohydrate	6 g
Dietary Fiber	1 g
Sugars	4 g
Protein	1 g

Tomato Sauté

4 Servings / Serving Size: 1/2 cup

2 tsp olive oil
3 scallions, minced
2 garlic cloves, minced
1 small red pepper, cored, seeded, and diced
2 cups cherry tomatoes, halved
2 large plum tomatoes, seeded and coarsely chopped
1 tsp sugar
1/2 tsp dried oregano
   Salt and pepper to taste
1 tsp lemon juice

1 Heat the oil in a large skillet over medium-high heat. Add the scallions and garlic and sauté for 2 minutes. Add the red pepper and sauté for 3 minutes.

2 Add the tomatoes, sugar, oregano, salt, and pepper and sauté for 3 minutes until the tomatoes begin to soften but still retain their shape. Add the lemon juice and serve.

Exchanges
2 Vegetable
1/2 Fat

Calories 59
  Calories from Fat . . . 24
Total Fat . . . . 3 g
  Saturated Fat . . . . . 0.3 g
Cholesterol . . . . 0 mg
Sodium . . . . 13 mg
Total Carbohydrate . . 9 g
  Dietary Fiber . . . . 2 g
  Sugars . . . . 6 g
Protein . . . . 1 g

Zucchini with Peppers and Tomatoes

4 Servings / Serving Size: about 1/2 cup

1 tsp olive oil
1 garlic clove, minced
2 medium zucchini, unpeeled, halved, and sliced
1 medium red pepper, seeded, cored, and sliced thin
1 cup cherry tomatoes, halved
2 tsp minced fresh oregano
   Salt and pepper to taste

1 Heat the oil in a large skillet over medium-high heat. Add the garlic and sauté for 30 seconds. Add the zucchini and sauté for 4 minutes. Add the red pepper and sauté for 2 minutes. Add the cherry tomatoes and oregano and sauté for 1 minute.

2 Cover and reduce the heat to low. Cook for 3 minutes more. Season with salt and pepper.

Exchanges
2 Vegetable

Calories 45
   Calories from Fat . . . 14
Total Fat . . . . 2 g
   Saturated Fat . . . . . 0.2 g
Cholesterol . . . . 0 mg
Sodium . . . . 14 mg
Total Carbohydrate . . 8 g
   Dietary Fiber . . . . 2 g
   Sugars . . . . 4 g
Protein . . . . 2 g

Fruit (Frutta)

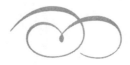

Five Ways with Fruit for Dessert: Italian Style

One of the things I love most about Italian cuisine is the deep appreciation for just capping off the meal lightly with fruit. Yes, of course, there are cannolis and other fancy confections, but I love the taste of fresh fruit enhanced with a drizzle of wine or freshly grated citrus zest. Here are some ideas for fruit that will end your meal on a delicious and healthy note!

Blueberries or Raspberries

1 Serving / Serving Size: 1/2 cup

For each 1/2 cup serving of berries, sprinkle with 1/4 tsp sugar and 1/4 tsp grated lemon zest and garnish with a sprig of fresh mint.

Exchanges
1 Fruit

Calories 45
  Calories from Fat . . . 2
Total Fat . . . . 0 g
  Saturated Fat . . . . . 0.0 g
Cholesterol . . . . 0 mg
Sodium . . . . 4 mg
Total Carbohydrate . 11 g
  Dietary Fiber . . . . 2 g
  Sugars . . . . 6 g
Protein . . . . 0 g

Melons

1 Serving / Serving Size: 1/4 melon

Sprinkle 1/2 tsp fresh lime juice and 1/4 tsp sugar on one quarter of a small honeydew or cantaloupe.

Exchanges
1 Fruit

Calories 46
  Calories from Fat 3
Total Fat . . . . 0 g
  Saturated Fat . . . . . 0.1 g
Cholesterol . . . . 0 mg
Sodium . . . . 11 mg
Total Carbohydrate . 11 g
  Dietary Fiber . . . . 1 g
  Sugars . . . . 10 g
Protein . . . . 1 g

Oranges

1 Serving / Serving Size: 1 orange

Peel and section one small orange
per person. Place the oranges in a
dessert bowl and drizzle each one
with 1 tsp Marsala wine. Cover and
refrigerate for a half hour before
serving.

Exchanges	
1 Fruit	

Calories 51	
Calories from Fat 1	
Total Fat . . . . 0 g	
Saturated Fat . . . . . 0.0 g	
Cholesterol . . . . 0 mg	
Sodium . . . . 0 mg	
Total Carbohydrate . 12 g	
Dietary Fiber . . . . 2 g	
Sugars . . . . 9 g	
Protein . . . . 1 g	

Peaches

1 Serving / Serving Size: 1/2 peach

Place half of a peeled and pitted
medium peach in a dessert dish.
Combine 2 Tbsp low-fat ricotta
cheese, 1/4 tsp sugar or sugar substitute, 1/4 tsp cinnamon, and a dash
of nutmeg. Stuff the peach with the
filling.

Exchanges	
1/2 Fruit	1/2 Fat

Calories 63	
Calories from Fat . . . 10	
Total Fat . . . . 1 g	
Saturated Fat . . . . . 1.0 g	
Cholesterol . . . . 12 mg	
Sodium . . . . 48 mg	
Total Carbohydrate . 10 g	
Dietary Fiber . . . . 1 g	
Sugars . . . . 8 g	
Protein . . . . 5 g	

Strawberries

1 Serving / Serving Size: 1/2 cup

Slice 1/2 cup of strawberries per serving. Sprinkle with 1/4 tsp sugar and 1 tsp of the very best balsamic vinegar you can afford. The taste contrast of sweet and slightly tart is amazing!

Exchanges
1/2 Fruit

Calories	32
Calories from Fat	3
Total Fat	0 g
Saturated Fat	0.0 g
Cholesterol	0 mg
Sodium	1 mg
Total Carbohydrate	8 g
Dietary Fiber	2 g
Sugars	6 g
Protein	1 g

Alphabetical List of Recipes

V

W

Z

Subject Index

A

Artichokes

Chicken with Artichokes, 52
Chicken with Italian Tomatoes and
    Artichokes, 55

Arugula

Arugula Salad, 130
Sautéed Arugula with Slivered
    Garlic, 150
Tuna on a Bed of Arugula, 21

Asparagus

Asparagus and Shrimp Pasta Toss, 97
Asparagus Salad, 131
Asparagus with Pine Nuts and Sun-
    Dried Tomatoes, 132
Fettuccine with Prosciutto and
    Asparagus, 100
Penne with Asparagus and Baby
    Spinach, 112
Roasted Asparagus, 148

B

Bacon

Orecchiette with Broccoli, Bacon,
    and Garlic, 106
Pork Cutlets with Bacon and Onions,
    83

Bass

Seared Bass with Basil, 15

Beans

Green Beans with Lemon, 141
Green Beans with Sautéed Onions,
    142
Green Beans with Tomatoes and
    Herbs, 143
Main Dish Tuscan Bean Salad, 125

Beef

Filet with Portobello Mushrooms,
    70
Garlic-Infused Beef Kebabs, 71
Sirloin Steak with Rosemary, 72
Steak Milanese, 73
Steak Pizzaiola, 74
Veal Marsala, 75
Veal Scallopini with Olives and Pine
    Nuts, 76
Veal with Leeks and Mushrooms,
    77
Veal with Leeks and Zucchini, 78
Veal with Sage and Garlic, 79

Broccoli

Broccoli with Lemon, 133
Broccoli with Red Onion and Pine
    Nuts, 134
Broccoli with Seasoned Walnuts,
    135
Fusilli with Broccoli, Peppers, and
    Asiago, 102
Garlicky Shrimp and Broccoli, 31
Orecchiette with Broccoli, Bacon,
    and Garlic, 106

C

Calamari

Shrimp and Calamari Salad, 39

Cauliflower

Cauliflower with Crumb Topping, 136

Cauliflower with Tomatoes and Peppers, 137

Pasta with Cauliflower, 108

Chicken

Balsamic Chicken and Tomato, 42

Balsamic Glazed Chicken, 43

Broiled Chicken Thighs with Basil and Pepper Sauce, 44

Chicken Cacciatore I, 45

Chicken Cacciatore II, 46

Chicken Cutlets with Garlic Plum Tomato Relish, 47

Chicken Cutlets with Sun-Dried Tomato Sauce, 48

Chicken in Balsamic Vinegar and Mustard, 49

Chicken Sauté with Lemon and Fennel, 50

Chicken Scallopini with Sage and Capers, 51

Chicken with Artichokes, 52

Chicken with Fresh Herbs and Shallots, 53

Chicken with Garlic Spinach, 54

Chicken with Italian Tomatoes and Artichokes, 55

Chicken with Peppers I, 56

Chicken with Peppers II, 57

Chicken with Porcini Mushrooms, 58

Chicken with Portobello Mushroom Sauce, 59

Chicken with Rosemary Sauce, 60

Chicken with Sage and Lemon, 61

Chicken with Shallot Sauce, 62

Easy Mediterranean-Style Chicken Salad, 63

Herb Grilled Chicken with Walnut Pesto, 64

Italian Chicken Salad with Walnuts, 65

Rosemary Lemon Chicken Thighs, 66

Rosemary Olive Chicken, 67

Clams

Linguine with Clams, 104

Cod

Baked Cod with Fresh Tomato Topping, 4

Cod with Grilled Tomatoes, 6

Cod with Oregano and Lemon, 7

Parsley- and Olive-Topped Cod, 11

E

Eggs

Frittata with Onion, 123

Zucchini Frittata, 126

F

Fennel

Chicken Sauté with Lemon and Fennel, 50

Fennel and Orange Salad, 138

Sautéed Fennel, 151

Fish. *See also* **Shellfish**

Baked Cod with Fresh Tomato Topping, 4

Broiled Tuna with Cherry Tomato Sauce, 5

Pork

Fettuccine with Prosciutto and
  Asparagus, 100
Orecchiette with Broccoli, Bacon,
  and Garlic, 106
Pancetta Penne, 107
Pork Chops with Sage and Rosemary,
  82
Pork Cutlets with Bacon and Onions,
  83
Pork Loin Chops with Herbed
  Mustard Sauce, 84
Pork Medallions with Pine Nuts and
  White Wine, 85
Pork Oreganata, 86
Pork Salad with Pine Nuts and Basil,
  87
Rigatoni with Pancetta, 115
Rosemary Pork Chops, 88
Sautéed Pork with Lemon and
  Parsley, 89
Whole Wheat Penne with
  Prosciutto, 120

Potatoes

Roasted Herb Potatoes, 149

Poultry. *See* Chicken

S

Salad

Arugula Salad, 130
Asparagus Salad, 131
Easy Mediterranean-Style Chicken
  Salad, 63
Fennel and Orange Salad, 138
Italian Chicken Salad with Walnuts,
  65
Main Dish Tuscan Bean Salad, 125

Pepper and Basil Salad, 146
Pork Salad with Pine Nuts and Basil,
  87
Shrimp and Basil Salad, 38
Shrimp and Calamari Salad, 39
Spinach Salad with Balsamic
  Dressing, 152
Tomato and Basil Salad, 154
Tuscan Tuna Salad, 27

Salmon

Grilled Salmon with Fresh Tomato
  Sauce, 9
Salmon in White Wine and Leeks, 12
Salmon with Fresh Tomato and
  Garlic Sauce, 13
Salmon with Lemon and Oregano, 14

Sandwiches

Hot Mushroom Open-Faced
  Sandwich, 124

Scallops

Herbed Scallops, 33
Lemon Scallops with Shallot Sauce,
  35
Scallops Florentine, 36
Seafood Mélange, 37

Shallots

Chicken with Fresh Herbs and
  Shallots, 53
Chicken with Shallot Sauce, 62
Lemon Scallops with Shallot Sauce,
  35

Shellfish. *See also* Fish

Angel Hair Pasta with Shrimp and
  Spinach, 96
Asparagus and Shrimp Pasta Toss, 97
Garlic Shrimp, 30

Garlicky Shrimp and Broccoli, 31
Grilled Parmigiana Shrimp over
 Sautéed Spinach, 32
Herbed Scallops, 33
Herbed Spicy Shrimp, 34
Lemon Scallops with Shallot Sauce,
 35
Linguine with Clams, 104
Scallops Florentine, 36
Seafood Mélange, 37
Shrimp and Basil Salad, 38
Shrimp and Calamari Salad, 39

Shrimp

Angel Hair Pasta with Shrimp and
 Spinach, 96
Asparagus and Shrimp Pasta Toss, 97
Garlic Shrimp, 30
Garlicky Shrimp and Broccoli, 31
Grilled Parmigiana Shrimp over
 Sautéed Spinach, 32
Herbed Spicy Shrimp, 34
Seafood Mélange, 37
Shrimp and Basil Salad, 38
Shrimp and Calamari Salad, 39

Sole

Marjoram-Flavored Sole Filets, 10

Spinach

Angel Hair Pasta with Shrimp and
 Spinach, 96
Chicken with Garlic Spinach, 54
Farfalle with Spinach and Cherry
 Tomatoes, 99
Grilled Parmigiana Shrimp over
 Sautéed Spinach, 32
Penne with Asparagus and Baby
 Spinach, 112

Spinach Salad with Balsamic
 Dressing, 152
Spinach with Garlic and Leeks, 153

Squash

Grated Zucchini and Yellow Squash
 Salad, 140
Grilled Zucchini and Yellow Squash
 Spears, 145

Swordfish

Fusilli and Swordfish, 101
Swordfish Sicilian Style, 17
Swordfish with Garlic and Parsley, 18

T

Tilapia

Tilapia in Zesty Tomato Sauce, 19

Tomatoes

Asparagus with Pine Nuts and Sun-
 Dried Tomatoes, 132
Baked Cod with Fresh Tomato
 Topping, 4
Balsamic Chicken and Tomato, 42
Broiled Tuna with Cherry Tomato
 Sauce, 5
Cauliflower with Tomatoes and
 Peppers, 137
Chicken Cutlets with Garlic Plum
 Tomato Relish, 47
Chicken Cutlets with Sun-Dried
 Tomato Sauce, 48
Chicken with Italian Tomatoes and
 Artichokes, 55
Cod with Grilled Tomatoes, 6
Farfalle with Spinach and Cherry
 Tomatoes, 99

Z

Zucchini

About the American Diabetes Association

The American Diabetes Association is the nation's leading voluntary health organization supporting diabetes research, information, and advocacy. Its mission is to prevent and cure diabetes and to improve the lives of all people affected by diabetes. The American Diabetes Association is the leading publisher of comprehensive diabetes information. Its huge library of practical and authoritative books for people with diabetes covers every aspect of self-care—cooking and nutrition, fitness, weight control, medications, complications, emotional issues, and general self-care.

To order American Diabetes Association books: Call 1-800-232-6733. Or log on to http://store.diabetes.org

To join the American Diabetes Association: Call 1-800-806-7801. www.diabetes.org/membership

For more information about diabetes or ADA programs and services: Call 1-800-342-2383. E-mail: AskADA@diabetes.org or log on to www.diabetes.org

To locate an ADA/NCQA Recognized Provider of quality diabetes care in your area: www.ncqa.org/dprp

To find an ADA Recognized Education Program in your area: Call 1-888-232-0822. www.diabetes.org/recognition/education.asp

To join the fight to increase funding for diabetes research, end discrimination, and improve insurance coverage: Call 1-800-342-2383. www.diabetes.org/advocacy

To find out how you can get involved with the programs in your community: Call 1-800-342-2383. See below for program Web addresses.

- *American Diabetes Month:* educational activities aimed at those diagnosed with diabetes—month of November. www.diabetes.org/ADM
- *American Diabetes Alert:* annual public awareness campaign to find the undiagnosed—held the fourth Tuesday in March. www.diabetes.org/alert
- *The Diabetes Assistance & Resources Program (DAR):* diabetes awareness program targeted to the Latino community. www.diabetes.org/DAR
- *African American Program:* diabetes awareness program targeted to the African American community. www.diabetes.org/africanamerican
- *Awakening the Spirit: Pathways to Diabetes Prevention & Control:* diabetes awareness program targeted to the Native American community. www.diabetes.org/awakening
- **To find out about an important research project regarding type 2 diabetes:** www.diabetes.org/ada/research.asp

To obtain information on making a planned gift or charitable bequest: Call 1-888-700-7029. www.diabetes.org/ada/plan.asp

To make a donation or memorial contribution: Call 1-800-342-2383. www.diabetes.org/ada/cont.asp